PENDULUMS AND THE LIGHT

Pendulums and the Light

Communication with the Goddess

Diane Stein

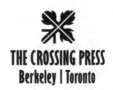

THE CROSSING PRESS
Berkeley | Toronto

The Crossing Press
A Division of Ten Speed Press
PO Box 7123
Berkeley, California 94707
www.tenspeed.com

Distributed in Australia by Simon and Schuster Australia, in Canada by Ten Speed
Press Canada, in New Zealand by Southern Publishers Group, in South Africa by
Real Books, and in the United Kingdom and Europe by Airlift Book Company.

Cover and text design by Lynn Bell, Monroe Street Studios

Library of Congress Cataloging-in-Publication Data
Stein, Diane, 1948–
Pendulums and the light : communication with the goddess / Diane Stein.
        p. cm.
Includes bibliographical references and index.
ISBN 1-58091-163-3 (pbk.)
1. Pendulum—Miscellanea. 2. Goddess religion. I. Title.
BF1628.3.S73   2004
204'.3—dc22   2004013701

Printed in the United States of America
First printing, 2004

1 2 3 4 5 6 7 8 9 10 — 09 08 07 06 05 04

FOR BREDE AND JESHUA
AND COMMUNICATION WITH THE LIGHT

CONTENTS

DIAGRAMS

WHY PENDULUMS?

For several years, people have been asking me to write a book on pendulums. My response has always been, "Pendulums don't need a book; they're so simple that anyone can use them. You can learn to use a pendulum in minutes." Recently, however, the requests to write this book have become more insistent and more frequent. So many of my Essential Energy Balancing students find using pendulums the easiest way to communicate with the Lords of Karma and their Goddesses, that I find myself teaching how to use a pendulum more and more often. It's become so often, in fact, that perhaps it really is time to write a book on pendulums and on using pendulums for karmic release and Goddess work.

Come to think of it, in my own early days of learning Women's Spirituality techniques, I found pendulum use very difficult. I had a friend who showed me how, and I bought a lovely short pendulum with a tumbled amethyst on the end, along with a very good how-to-do-it pamphlet, at the Michigan Women's Music Festival. Yet, as often as I was shown how and as much as I read the pamphlet and other books, I couldn't seem to get the pendulum to work for me. I went again and again to my friend, who couldn't understand why I couldn't learn this simple technique and who was getting very tired of me calling every time I had a question I needed a pendulum to answer.

The pendulum wasn't working for me for a variety of reasons. I couldn't read the "yes" and "no" swings it was making. It was swinging in a circle for both "yes" and "no," the difference being in the direction of the swing. My lack of depth perception made it impossible for me to tell the difference in the swing directions. In addition, the chain from which the amethyst hung was too short, stiff, and thick to be comfortable for me—with a longer, thinner chain and the accompanying freer swing, I would have been able to read the responses. The chain was also of a cheap mixed metal that didn't transmit energy very well, and its motions were sloppy and irregular. I had no idea of how or why to keep a pendulum energetically cleared, especially one made with gemstones. I didn't know that an uncleared pendulum cannot be accurate. In addition, it didn't occur to me to dedicate my pendulum to the Light or to ask my Goddess (or any other Light-being, spirit guide, angel, or Higher Self) to work through it. I also didn't know the most important pendulum skill—how to phrase the questions for optimal response.

Pendulums didn't work for me until I learned these things and more. While the methods and "rules" are simple and should be common sense, they weren't so for me and probably aren't for others new to using this tool. Gradually, I learned how to choose or make pendulums that worked for me, pendulums with the best materials for optimal use, the right chain or string length, and the perfect weight of the swinging pendant at the end. I learned how to dedicate pendulums, to clear them and keep them clear, and to make sure that only Be-ings of the Highest Light were permitted to communicate through them. I learned who some of those Be-ings are and why they choose to work with us. And I learned how to ask questions in a way that would give me reliably accurate responses every time.

As I learned these skills by trial and error, the pendulum became an increasingly important and useful tool in my healing and energy work. I began to stretch the limits of what a pendulum could do, and I began to do things like psychic readings, healing, and karmic work with them. Friends laughed at me for these uses, assuring me that I couldn't be accurate and that pendulums "say anything you want them to." I had learned how to do better than that, and gradually the scoffers stopped scoffing and wanted to know how I did it.

When the more than planetary karmic work I was doing became psychically dangerous, the Lords of Karma and Divine Director shut off my psychic hearing for a time, the ability I have always depended upon totally. They did it for my protection and for the protection of my Goddess Brede. To do the Lightwork I was meant to do, I then had to find another means of communication, and the pendulum became that means. Now, even with my psychic hearing restored, using a pendulum has its frequent place. Pendulum use requires less psychic concentration than using clairaudience/psychic hearing and is a useful alternative on many occasions.

I have a pendulum in my hand, or close by and ready, at all times. When not in use, which is seldom, it is in a small pouch in my pocket. I keep a pendulum on my nightstand when I go to bed; by my side while reading, writing, or studying; and at the ready while shopping, healing, gardening, talking on the phone, teaching, doing psychic work, dealing with the bank or auto mechanic, and for virtually everything else that I do day or night. I keep more than a dozen pendulums clearing under a pyramid on my bedroom Goddess altar; changing them frequently, I use several different pendulums each day. I have learned to make my own pendulums, to my own specifications, and make dozens of them in a wide variety of materials.

I used to be embarrassed when someone would see me using a pendulum in the bookstore, supermarket, or health food store. I've long since gotten over this discomfort, since the value of having the tool in these and every other situation far outweighs any embarrassment. Occasionally a stranger wants to know what "that thing" is. Sometimes I show them, and sometimes I just tell them it's a "worry stone." If a shopkeeper pressures me about it, I will sooner stop buying at that store than stop using the pendulum. It is just too valuable. I once told an obnoxious store owner to "Mind your own business if you want mine!" He did, and I made my purchase—guided by the pendulum and the Light-being communicating with me through it. Come to think of it, there are lots of reasons to write a book about pendulums and the Goddess.

A pendulum, a tool as simple as a button on a string with a capability for only a "yes" or "no" response, has an endless variety of uses in psychic work and in daily life. The accuracy of its use depends upon your ability to connect to a Goddess or other Be-ing of the Light to work through it. (The how-to is discussed beginning in chapter four.) That done, its binary code, "yes" or "no," becomes a rudimentary computer whose limits are only bound by your imagination and your ability to ask the right questions (also discussed in chapter seven). Once you learn your way around this psychic tool, you will have it in your hand all the time as I do, and will wonder how you ever did without it.

A pendulum can be used for energy diagnostics to determine what is wrong with anything, from a car to your own body. You can use it in your home to estimate what a repair will cost and to determine the origin of the problem or dis-ease. To do this, you need to ask "yes" or "no" questions of the Light-being running the tool. If she doesn't know, she will find a Be-ing who can get you accurate responses. Your questions have to be phrased simply, with an unambiguous "yes" or "no" as the only possible answer. For example, you can ask about your malfunctioning car, "Is the problem the battery?" If the answer is "no," what else could it be? "Is the problem the alternator?" This is a "yes." Then your next request might be to find out what it will cost to fix it. You might ask, "Will it cost less than $100?" If the answer is "no," ask, "Will it cost less than $150?" And so on in increasing amounts (you can use less or more) until you get a "yes."

The possibilities for pendulum use are endless. Of two jobs you are interviewing for, which job would bring the most satisfaction? Phrase the request something like, "Would Job A be the most positive employment for me?" "Would Job B?" "Would both be equally positive?" (Or equally negative?) "Would Job A bring the most money?" "Would Job B pay better?" "Will I be offered one of these jobs?" "Will I be offered both?" "Will I be offered neither?" "Is it more positive for me to accept Job A?" "Is it more positive for me to accept Job B?" "Would I get along well with the boss at Job A?" "Would I get along well with the boss at Job B?" "Should I make my application today?" Or, "Would it be best to wait until tomorrow?" "Should I call?" "Is this dress the best one to wear on the first day of the new job?"

In relationships, the pendulum questions are similar. "Should I ask her for a date?" "Is there potential for a love relationship with this person?" "Is the person I'm considering moving in with a compatible mate for me?" "Will the relationship last longer than a year?" "Will it last longer than ten years?" "Is this my life mate?" "Will I be happy in a relationship or marriage with this person?" Be very sure you have a Goddess or Light-being working through your pendulum before you ask serious life questions, and be very confident that your pendulum work is accurate before you place trust in the answers. If your own knowing disagrees with the pendulum, and you are not fully confident in who is communicating with you, trust your own knowing first. If your knowing disagrees, and you *are* confident in your angel, spirit guide, or Goddess, ask further questions to reconcile the discrepancy. Usually the answer is in how you frame your questions.

In finding a place to live, your pendulum questions might go something like the following: "Is this ad for an apartment worth following up on?" "Would I be happy living in this place?" "Are there discarnate spirits [ghosts] that need to be passed over here?" If so, "Are they in the house or apartment?" "Are they in other apartments or rooms of the building?" "Are they in the yard or somewhere on the grounds?" "Are there energies in this apartment or house that are not of the Light?" "Can the Light-being running this pendulum clear the energy and remove the discarnate spirit, taking it to where it properly belongs?" "Will you do it now?" "Is there more that I need to know?" "Once this is done and the energy is cleared, should I sign a lease to live here?" Always remember to say "please" and "thank you" to the guide, Goddess, angel, or Light-being who is running the pendulum to communicate with you and help you. Do this always and without exception.

There are any number of questions that a Light-being or Goddess running your pendulum can answer, and answer with positive guidance. In any situation where there is choice, and you can't decide between choices, a pendulum is valuable. Ask which dentist or chiropractor you should chose, practitioner A or B, and if you need a dentist or chiropractor at all. This question would actually be three separate questions asked one at a time. The three questions are "Do I need a practitioner at this time at all?" "Should I go to Practitioner A?" "Should I go to practitioner B?" A further question might be, "Is there a practitioner C that might be better than both A and B?" Ask further questions to locate that practitioner.

A pendulum can be used to find lost objects. Start by asking, "Are my keys still in the house?" If "yes," then list the rooms of your house one by one, asking with each room's name, "Are my missing keys in the kitchen?" If "no," ask, "Are they in the living room?" And so on, until you get a "yes." Go to the room where the pendulum says they should be. If you can't see the keys, ask, "Are they under something?" If "no," ask, "Are they in a drawer?" If this is "yes," list the drawers until you get another "yes" and look in that drawer. You might also ask, "Are they there *now?*" A Goddess or angel has no sense of time; all time is the present to her. If the keys were there yesterday but are not there today, you might get a "yes" unless you are specific.

A friend called me on the phone frantic because she couldn't find her kitten. She thought the cat couldn't have gotten out, but maybe she had. She hadn't seen her in at least an hour and there was nowhere in her small duplex a kitten could hide. The door hadn't been opened for the cat to go outside; it was an indoor cat and very young, afraid of the outdoors. I took out a pendulum and started asking, room by room, which room the white kitten was in. By a series of questions, the information was that the cat was in the kitchen "inside something," but Carolyn couldn't see her. Food offers didn't bring her out. My friend opened the lower cupboard doors and found the kitten inside one of them, asleep on a shelf surrounded by cooking pots and wondering what the fuss was all about.

I once was asked to find a quantity of money that a man who had died in an auto accident had put away for emergencies. His widow needed the money for the funeral expenses, knew it was in their home or garage, but couldn't find it. By process of elimination with the pendulum, the money had to be in one of the four shelf drawers on the garage's far wall. The woman searched there, but the drawers were empty of cash. The money was finally found in an envelope in the deceased man's pocket. No one knew why it was there when he had had the auto accident that killed him. His widow later told me that the drawer my pendulum indicated, in a house I had never been in, was where he had normally kept the funds.

I also like to use pendulums for driving directions. Do this only when you know where you're headed but have to make simple choices about how to get there. Don't use a pendulum to drive somewhere if you have no idea where you're going; this is a tool for fine-tuning. (People riding in the car with me tend to not trust it and are always surprised when it works.) Be very careful using pendulums or any other psychic ability or tool while driving, since you may be in a deeper meditative or focused state than you realize and could put yourself and others in danger. Pull off and stop before bringing out the pendulum. (Do as I say, not as I do!) Before getting into the car, you can hold your pendulum over a map to help you determine the quickest route with the least traffic. You can also ask about your route with a series of questions, without a map, before leaving home. Again, remember that you have to phrase your questions very simply, since your answers are only "yes" or "no."

In the same way, it is possible to ask when something will happen or be completed. "Will I receive my paycheck tomorrow?" "Will the handyman show up today?" In asking time questions, realize that for Lightbeings not in body all time is now and pinpointing a particular increment of Earth time can be difficult for them. Some are better at doing this accurately than others. Also realize that when you ask a time question, you will get the answer *as it is at this moment*. If something changes five minutes from now, the answer will no longer be accurate. For example, if the handyman was heading your way but got an emergency call to delay him, the answer that was correct before he got the call will no longer be correct once he's been sidetracked. You can ask if something will happen by a particular time but also specify the day. "Will the handyman come by three o'clock?" "Will he come *today* by three o'clock?" In using a pendulum for time questions, there are a number of variables, and these questions tend to be the least accurate—and the most frustrating—of pendulum uses.

Pendulums are also important healing tools, and if time is their weakness, healing is where they usually have the greatest accuracy. They can be used to discover which chakra is out of alignment, whether a chakra is too closed or too open, and to locate and assess areas where there is or has been dis-ease. They can be used to analyze your choices for healing the imbalances you discover—which crystal or gemstone will help, which healing method is useful for the situation (Reiki, laying on of hands, gemstones, aura stroking, herbs, and so forth). You can use a pendulum to help you choose a homeopathic remedy, herb, or vitamin supplement for your needs, and you can ask a pendulum which nutrients you may be deficient in. If you suspect allergies, you can determine whether you are sensitive to a food, soap, chemical, or any other substance in this way as well.

If you are able to hold the nutrient or remedy bottle in your hand while asking, your responses will be more precise. Brede tells me that She knows many substances by their vibrations, rather than by their names, and gets more information for me when I touch what I'm asking about. Do this to determine remedy dosages. Hold the remedy or herb package in the hand not holding the pendulum and ask how many drops or capsules you need per dose or per day. Hold the pendulum as you count from "one" upward. You will get a "yes" response when you reach the correct number. Also ask how many times per day to take the dose. You can usually determine how long you will need to take the remedy as well, all by phrasing your questions for "yes" or "no" answers with your pendulum. As you can see from the examples of this chapter, a pendulum is almost limitless in its uses.

An extremely important use of pendulums, which will be covered more thoroughly in chapter eleven, is using the pendulum for working with the Lords of Karma for karmic release and healing. This is just one more of many pendulum uses, but it's a use you will find extremely valuable. Even if your psychic abilities are undeveloped and you don't think you are psychic, you will be amazed at the communication you can achieve through the simple pendulum. Work with the Lords of Karma is always life changing and life affirming. For more information on karma and karmic release, see my books on the subject: *We Are the Angels, Essential Energy Balancing, Reliance on the Light, Essential Energy Balancing II,* and *Essential Energy Balancing III* (forthcoming). Most of today's karmic healing issues can be cleared quickly, easily, and immediately in this lifetime. This is a great gift offered to us by the Lords of Karma and our Great Mother Nada—one of the greatest gifts we on Earth have ever received. It's something to make the best use of that you can, in every way that you can.

A little background on pendulum origins is in order here. Though used in modern Goddess, Wiccan, and New Age spirituality, pendulums are not new and they have a long herstory as healing tools. Dowsing is the old-time term for employing a variety of pendulums and pendulum-type implements (called "dowsers"), usually for finding hidden things. Such tools include dowsing rods, y-rods, witching sticks, large long-string pendulums or plumb bobs, and a tool known as a "bobber," all of which work on the same principles as modern pendulums. They were traditionally used for the non-spiritual purposes of locating underground water, so drinking wells could be dug, and for finding minerals and metals in commercial mining. More recently, such tools and dowsing are used to locate the underground water of geopathic zones, places of potentially negative energy that form under some homes and buildings. Once found, these zone energies can be deflected, making the houses above them healthy again.

References to dowsing in art and literature go back as far as eight thousand years ago and are worldwide. Pendulums and dowsing tools were known in central Africa, India, Sweden, Denmark, Malaysia, Polynesia,

Peru, and pre-Contact America. Records go back to biblical times of pendulums and dowsing by Hebrews, Egyptians, Scythians, Persians, Medes, and Etruscans. They were known to the Greeks and Romans of classical times and were used by the Celtic Druids and the ancient Chinese. The following brief survey comes from a variety of books on dowsing; see the suggested reading list at the end of this book for more information on dowsing in early cultures.

The earliest known reference to dowsing and pendulums is dated at 6000 B.C.E. In the Tassili Caves in southern Algeria, four pictographs of human figures, one of which is holding a y-rod, were discovered in 1949. In China in 2200 B.C.E., Emperor Yu was known as a dowser and explorer and is believed to have sailed ships to the western United States and Mexican coasts. He left written decrees forbidding the building of homes on geopathic zones, and such zones were located even then by dowsing. Much later, Venetian Marco Polo knew and used pendulums, dowsing rods, and the compass, and he learned of them in China. He traveled there from 1271 to 1295.

In the Old Testament (Numbers 20:8–11), Moses and Aaron used a rod to find water in the desert. In the Exodus from Egypt, Moses' rod became a serpent and also held back the waters of the Nile for the Hebrews to cross. There are frequent mentions of dowsing in the Old Testament, which was probably written down around 1300 B.C.E.Egyptian hieroglyphic writings of the biblical era describe a magician's wand or rod that was also a dowsing rod, called Ur-Heka, which meant "great magical power [that] makes water to come forth."[1] The Queen of Sheba is mentioned in the Old Testament as a user of dowsing for prophecy, and it is said that King Solomon used dowsing to choose women for his harem. The later Queen Cleopatra, who was eighteen years old when she came to power in Egypt at around 47 B.C.E., was said to have dowsers with her at all times. Dowsing rods operate slightly differently from pendulums but are closely related and are used in the same ways for the same purposes. They are the forerunners of today's small swinging pendulums.

In more recent times, the Spanish Inquisition (formally from 1478 to 1834, but actually in effect at least a century earlier) resulted in the deaths of millions of women as Witches. Many were accused and died because they were dowsers. There were also Witchcraft trials in the colonial United States, where dowsing was universally used to find water for drinking and crop irrigation. Dowsing for water is still called "water witching," and a raw forked tree branch sometimes used for dowsing is called a "witching stick." The Inquisition attempted to eradicate Goddess religion and women's psychic and healing abilities, and dowsing was an evident use of both. Nine million people, almost all of them women and girls, were burned at the stake or hung in the years of the Inquisition. Most were tortured before they died. They were Goddess worshippers, psychics, healers, herbalists, dowsers, and midwives.

In 1518, Martin Luther, the founder of Protestantism, declared that using the rod was a violation of the First Commandment ("Thou shalt have no other Gods before Me"). Interestingly, Luther was the son of a miner, and the mining industry of the time frequently used dowsing to locate metals and minerals. There are many mentions of dowsing and pendulum use in German literature from the twelfth to fifteenth centuries, in the same period that women were being burned at the stake for being dowsers. Queen Elizabeth I of England (1558 to 1603) brought German dowsers to Cornwall to aid local miners in finding tin deposits.

By 1600, despite the persecutions, dowsing as a mining practice was very much in use throughout Europe. Though highly successful and lucrative, dowsing was still suspect. In 1627 in France, Martine de Berthereau and her husband, Baron de Beausoleil et d'Auffenbach, were sentenced to life in prison for Witchcraft. Martine was highly skilled as a dowser from a very young age and had located underground coal deposits that resulted in the opening and operation of more than 150 profitable coal mines. She was rewarded only with ingratitude. She and her husband were later released but all their equipment was confiscated. Martine de Berthereau became Mining Advisor to the French

Government, a position unheard of for a woman. By dowsing, she discovered the Chateau-Thierry mineral springs in 1629.

In 1640, de Berthereau published a book on dowsing and dowsing instruments called *La restitution de pluton*. Both authorship and publication were quite unusual for women of her day. She and her husband were arrested for Witchcraft again, and they died in separate prisons. It is interesting to note that in 1701, the use of dowsing to track criminals was outlawed in France. Criminal tracking was probably done with pendulums, rather than rods, as pendulums for dowsing were in use by this time, and such dowsing was apparently common practice.[2]

Dowsing with pendulums and rods went into decline in the 1800s, because in this supposed Age of Reason no one could explain how or why they worked. The great physicist Albert Einstein (1879–1955) was interested in dowsing and was a dowser himself. He predicted that science would one day have explanations for the phenomenon. Sir Isaac Newton, Leonardo da Vinci, and Thomas Edison were all scientists who were dowsers. The nineteenth century's extreme rationalism and denial of what it could not explain have prevailed in the arrogance of current established thought.

Pendulum techniques were revived in the 1920s in England when Medical Radiesthesia was developed as a healing field. An outgrowth of pendulum use and dowsing, radionics machines (basically complicated dowsing rods or pendulums) were developed, and many medical doctors of the time adopted them. (Today in the United States, this is an embattled science, though a valid one. True to form, the Food and Drug Administration confiscates such machines whenever it finds them. I have experienced them and they work.) Pendulums, rather than dowsing rods, came into popular use at this time also, especially for use in medical diagnostics. More than twenty-five hundred medical doctors in France used pendulums for diagnosis, and the trend continued until after World War II.

There was a world resurgence in every form of spirituality from the end of World War I through World War II, especially in France, England, and the United States. So many people died at war that seances in which mediums channeled messages from the dead became highly popular. Early modern investigation of Ascension processes and the Lords of Karma were begun at this time as well.

Pendulums and dowsing have been used by armies worldwide, beginning with the ancient Greeks. During World War II, General George Patton employed dowsers, as did Secretary of State Robert McNamara in the Vietnam War. In Vietnam, they were used to locate land mines, ammunition dumps, and underground tunnels.[3] In the 1960s, Soviet geologists also revived dowsing as a successful mining experiment. The Soviets were quite interested in psychic phenomena and tried to harness them for Cold War espionage. They didn't succeed, but their trying revived world interest in the scientific investigation of psychic abilities and made these abilities "respectable " once more. A number of modern corporations worldwide are noted by Greg Nielsen and Joseph Polansky in their book *Pendulum Power* for employing dowsers using rods or pendulums for a variety of purposes.[4]

And so we come to the present. Pendulums and related dowsing tools have a long and distinguished record of worldwide use and sometimes a record of poor treatment of their users. Today's primary dowsing tool is the simple weight-dangling-from-a-chain pendulum that anyone can learn to use. The uses of this simple tool go beyond mining and industry and into spirituality and healing, psychic ability, and clairvoyance, Goddess work, karmic release—and so much more.

How to Make or Buy a Pendulum

All kinds of small objects, dangling from a variety of cords, threads, strings, or chains can be used as pendulums. Pendulums can be bought in stores or easily made at home. There are many different styles of pendulums available, with a number of possibilities as to materials, weight, size, length, quality, and cost. Pendulums can be extremely beautiful or simply utilitarian; they can be ugly or just plain silly (and even the silly ones work quite well). They can be made of natural or synthetic materials, plastics or metals, crystals or wood. Some aspects of form and materials affect the accuracy and function of a pendulum, while others do not. Imagination and fancy can have full play for the creative—or you can pick something from a hardware or fishing store, New Age store, or bead store.

First let's look at some of the simplest pendulums, things to pick up and use when you need, on the spur of the moment, a spiritually guided answer. Some of these things can be used only once, for they won't last longer. A pendulum by definition is a free-swinging weight at the end of a short cord or chain. The length can vary from about four inches to a foot, according to your choice. When people ask me what they need to make a pendulum, I tell them, "Anything, even a button on a string." Take a small button and use a needle and thread to sew the thread through two of the buttonholes. Leaving the doubled thread about eight inches long, remove the needle and knot the thread at the top. You now have a beginning pendulum. If you are already familiar with pendulum work, try using it.

There are lots of small swinging objects that can be made into or used as is for a beginning pendulum. I say "beginning" because once you start using this tool, you will want more sophisticated models made with materials that transmit energy more strongly than plastic and thread. You will want pendulums that won't fall apart after the first use and that can become your permanent companions. For now, though, try a few more of the beginning versions. Take the needle and thread again, and stab the point of the needle into the center of a wine cork. Insert it fairly deeply. Take the doubled thread and knot it at the top, and you have another type of "found" pendulum. Compare the weight and swing of this pendulum, which will probably be heavier than the button and thread one you made before. Which feels more comfortable to use? Which feels more solid and has a more readable swing? Hold the string at various lengths to see what is the most comfortable for you.

Try a large paperclip with thread strung through it for your next "found" pendulum. How does the motion of this compare to the previous two? Try a small Christmas ball or ornament, putting a thread or thin string through the hanging loop, and see how these compare to the other examples. Try a teabag, swinging the bag from the attached cord and tag; try using it both dry and wet, and see which you prefer. Compare each of these throwaway pendulum types with the others. Which do you like or dislike? Which feels better to hold? Why? If you are already working with pendulums, try asking questions using each of these constructions. Do some work better than others?

You will find that heavier weights work better than lighter ones and that the freer the weight swings on the string the easier it is to use. By experiment, you will find your optimal string length and discover that you prefer one kind of string or cord over others. Do you like to hold your pendulum close to the weight or to use a longer string for a wider motion? Are some types of these "found" pendulums more accurate in their information than other types? Some materials seem inert, giving no answers at all, while others seem so active as to feel almost alive.

Many objects that you usually carry with you can be used for pendulums as well. Try swinging your key ring and bunch of keys, and ask for guided information. If you have a key ring with a single key on it, try that too. If you can make the keys swing, the pendulum will work. Try taking a key from the ring and threading a piece of string a few inches long through it or swinging it from a necklace chain. If you happen to have the kind of key used to turn antique lamps on and off, make that into a pendulum. Ask some "yes" and "no" questions with these arrangements and see how they work as pendulums. Again, notice which work and which don't, which you like best and least, and be aware of why.

Now try some hardware store or toolbox objects. Find a metal nut (the kind that fits onto a screw), put a doubled length of string or thread through it, and try it as a pendulum. The pendulum should hang and dangle at least four or five inches (and up to twelve inches) from the top of the string. Again, in all of the pendulums that you make, try varied string lengths until you find the length that is most comfortable for you. Make different pendulums using a shiny stainless steel nut, a brass nut, a dull-finished nickel one, a copper one, and a plastic one. Try something made of lead. Make each into a simple pendulum, and compare how they feel to use, how well they swing, and what your response with them is when you use them to ask for guidance. Look for other toolbox objects that a string or cord can pass through, and try them in the same way. You can use metal washers, for example, of several different sizes, materials, and weights.

Also from the hardware store, notice the types of weights that are available in the fishing department. These either have a hole through them or a loop at the top for tying them onto a fishing rod. They come in various sizes and materials. Experiment with a few. If there is a loop at the top, use them in the same way that you used the previous objects. Thread a piece of string through the loop, knot the string at the top, and test the swing. If they have a hole all the way through the object, you will need to thread the string through the weight, tying it at the bottom with a knot large enough to prevent the string from pulling through. This will take a heavier piece of cord or string, even a leather thong. Experiment with them.

How do the different materials compare? These are heavier weights than you've used before, and you may like them better. The shiny brass weights can make attractive pendulums. The duller lead fishing weights are less attractive, and they generally do not make good psychic tools. Lead doesn't transmit energy. While in the hardware store, look at the plumbing supplies. You may find there a plumbing bob, a relatively large metal or wooden point-ended cylinder with a ring or loop at the top. These bobs can be as much as nine inches long. They are sometimes used in dowsing and were the earliest type of swinging pendulums developed. Try them. You will need a longer and thicker string to use with these, or a length of medium chain, heavy enough that so large a weight doesn't cause it to break. How does it feel to work with something so big?

If you wear a necklace on any type of fine jewelry chain, open the clasp and take it off. Use the pendant on the necklace as your pendulum weight, and hold the doubled chain at a comfortable length in your dominant hand. Test this pendulum by asking a few "yes" or "no" questions with it. How to use a pendulum follows later in this book; you may skip ahead and read chapter six now if you are new to pendulum use. As a reader of this book, however, you may be already using pendulums. Experiment with these found objects for accuracy. If your necklace chain has no dangling pendant on it, take off a ring you may be wearing and string the chain through that. The ring dangling from the doubled chain also becomes a pendulum. Again, notice how the swing feels, and if you are already using pendulums to ask questions with, try this version for comfort and accuracy. Compare these forms of "found" pendulums with the flimsier teabag and button and the clumsier keys. I would be very surprised if you didn't prefer the necklace with the pendant or ring.

If you are lucky enough to have a holey stone, try it as a pendulum. These are small grey or brown stones found on beaches, with a natural hole through them. The stones are generally less than two inches in size, flat, and with irregular holes about half the size of a dime through them. Legend has it that if you look through a holey stone, you'll see fairies and nature spirits. Another legend says that if you look at the world through a holey stone, you will see only truth. Some Green Witches (who work with and in nature) wear them as necklace pendants. Make a pendulum of one of these stones by stringing a thin leather thong through the hole, knotting it at the top, and swinging the stone to use in asking your questions. You may decide that this is the pendulum you are looking for.

You are now at the point of making a permanent pendulum of your own. By this time, you know what you like, what feels good and is the most comfortable to use, and what is the most responsive when you ask for guidance. You know what length of thread or chain is the most comfortable to hold and which materials seem to work best. By example, here are my own preferences, which may be very different from yours. I like weights made of a crystal or gemstone point or pendant, or a heavier solid brass pointed weight (which has the added advantage of being unbreakable). Both are usually about an inch in length and no more than half an inch in diameter. Some brass pendulum weights are beautifully shaped. I like semi-thin necklace chain (usually silver) to swing the pendant on, and my chains are shorter than usual (three or four inches). I also like to have a bead at the top of the chain for holding the pendulum.

Aesthetics are important to me. A pendulum that is a brass weight or a crystal is very attractive. The brass weight can be silver plated and therefore silver in color, or it can be the gold-toned brass. A crystal or gemstone pendant usually has a silver or silver-colored mounting, and I choose chain in a color to match. The bead at the top is generally a gemstone bead that is the same kind of stone as the pendant (if gemstone or crystal). My metal pendant will also have a colored gemstone bead on the end of the chain to hold it. A disadvantage of gemstone and crystal pendants is their fragility. My pendulums receive hard use, and I frequently drop them. Crystal pendants shatter, and I need to replace them more often than I like to; metal pendants are unbreakable but are also less available to buy.

Now that you know what you want for a pendulum and have experimented and at least begun to learn to use one, the next step is to find or make yours. You can buy a pendulum or continue the experiments above, and with a few simple jewelry-making tips, you can easily learn to make your own. You also need to know that most people who work frequently with pendulums have more than one of them. Pendulums have to be kept energetically cleared to be accurate and can only be used for a couple of hours before they require cleansing. Since I need many pendulums, I make my own. If I were to buy them all, it would become expensive very quickly. You can probably make a dozen at home for what it costs to buy one in a store or from a catalog. If you have a variety of pendulums, some will become favorites, and in using them you will fine-tune your criteria for what you need.

If you make your own pendulums, you will need some jewelry-making tools and findings (jump rings, head pins, and so on), in addition to the pendants, chains, and beads. The tools are inexpensive and can be found in bead stores, jewelry-making catalogs, and craft shops. Of the catalogs, Fire Mountain Gems is my favorite (www.firemountaingems.com or (800) 423-2319), and there are many others. Catalog shopping for findings will be much less expensive than buying from bead stores, and catalogs have better quality materials than the craft shops carry. Look at a copy of *Lapidary Journal,* a magazine you can find in larger bookstores, for a variety of jewelry supply sources. Bead stores or jewelry-making catalogs also offer chains, beads, and pendants, and they often offer specially designed pendulum ends. Pendants and pendulum ends can also be purchased at New Age stores (as can finished pendulums in various types and prices). You might want to attend local gem and jewelry shows, which sell findings, chain, pendants, beads, and finished pendulums— along with much more.

The two jewelry-making tools you'll need are a forming tool called rosary pliers and flat-nose or chain nose pliers. The rosary pliers have rounded ends for bending wire into a loop and also are a cutting tool for the thin jewelry wire you will use. The flat-nose or chain-nose pliers are a smaller and more delicate version of ordinary pliers. They are used to bend thin metal and close jump rings, and they have a thousand uses. There are more expensive brands of these tools, but you should be able to buy both for about ten dollars. If you can buy both the chain-nose and flat-nose pliers, giving you three tools instead of two, you will be glad you did.

You will also need findings—jump rings and head pins. Jump rings are small (get about the 5mm size), thin, metal open rings that you will close in the process of making your pendulum. Be sure to buy jump rings, not split rings or soldered rings. Packages of jump rings sell for under three dollars for a hundred pieces in plated silver or plated gold. If you want pure silver or gold, you will pay more, but the greater expense is usually unnecessary. Use one of these rings to connect the pendulum chain to the loop at the top of the pendulum weight. Hook the chain end and pendulum loop onto the jump ring, then use the flat-nose or chain-nose pliers to gently bend the ring closed. If you hold one pair of pliers in each hand to twist the ring closed, you will get the best results.

When it is closed properly, the jump ring joining feels smooth when you run your finger over it, and the circle is complete with no overlap. A gap in the ring allows your chain or pendulum end to fall off, while an overlap prevents the chain or pendant from moving freely and hampers the pendulum's swing. With practice, you will learn to close the rings properly (and there is even a tool available to do it with, if you wish).

The other finding you will need is called a head pin. Head pins also come in precious or semiprecious types, and the silver-plated or gold-plated are fine. Head pins look like straight pins for sewing, but without the sharp point. They are longer and are made of metal soft enough to be bent and formed into a loop. Head pins come in a variety of lengths, and the one-and-a-half-inch size is probably the most useful for your purpose. They also come in two thicknesses, .021 inch thick and .028 inch. The .021-inch size is of thinner metal, which fits through smaller beads that have smaller holes. The thinner pins are easier to bend and shape, but thinner also means that they wear out and break more easily. The .028-inch pins are sturdier but are too thick to fit through the drilling of many beads. Since they cost about three dollars for a package of a hundred, you may wish to buy both sizes. Eye pins are similar to head pins, except that instead of a straight-pin-like head at the end they have a small loop.

You will use a head pin to put a loop on the end of a bead so that you can connect it either directly to the pendulum chain or to a jump ring between the bead and the chain. You will also use a head pin on a pendulum weight that has no metal mounting (no loop end) but that has a hole drilled through it. In both cases, the pin goes through the hole, leaving part of the pin sticking out from the bead or pendant. Take your rosary pliers and, using the cutting side, first cut the pin so that just slightly more than half an inch of it is still protruding from the bead or pendulum weight. Grip the bead or weight with your other hand.

Then with the rounded jaws of the rosary pliers, clamp the middle of the remaining pin and pull it gently toward you, while at the same time rotating the pliers (and wire) down and away from you. The round end of the pliers will make a round bend in the pin wire. Continue bending the wire on the rosary pliers until you have a rounded loop. Use your wrist for the motion. Hook your chain over the resulting loop, and use your rosary pliers or chain-nose pliers to close the loop. If you use a jump ring to connect the new loop on the bead to the chain, it will make a nicer finish. Your bead will be connected solidly to the chain, and it will be able to move freely. If your pendulum pendant requires a head pin, do it the same way.

The job of making a pendulum takes only a few minutes, and it is harder and slower to explain it than to do it. If you have a bead store in your area, get someone there to show you. Once you've seen it, you'll have it down. Most pendulum pendants come with a loop already on the end, and with these you will not need the head pin. It only takes a jump ring to connect the pendulum end to the chain. On the other hand, if you want a bead at the top, few beads come with the loop already finished. After a few tries, you'll do it easily yourself. The bead at the end is optional, but it makes holding the pendulum far more comfortable. Choose a bead that is not too large, probably an 8mm or 10mm bead is the largest you'll want. Unless you buy very expensive pendulum pendants, it should not cost more than a couple of dollars to make a pendulum, once you have the findings. And don't forget that the hardware nut or washer on a string still works.

In summary, there are a variety of materials from which you can make a beautiful and optimally functioning pendulum. Pointed brass pendulum ends—available at gem shows and from jewelry-making catalogs, bead shops, and New Age stores—are probably the best. They come with a loop on the end, so you do not need head pins. Second best, in my opinion, are clear crystal pendants, which you can find in the same places. Next, after clear crystal points, I like colored gemstone pendants. They are best when pointed on the end, either as flat-faceted gemstone points or cylinder shaped with a pointed end. If you find them in these forms, they will also already have the attaching loop. Many pendulum users prefer wooden pendants in the pointed cylinder shape. Some of these in polished woods can be extremely beautiful, and they carry energy well. The issue here, besides your personal choice of aesthetics, is to find the materials that will best transmit psychic energy. Most pendulum users prefer natural materials, whether of stone, wood, or metal. Again, plastic and synthetic materials don't carry energy well, and lead doesn't carry energy at all.

Your choice of pendulum chain is also important, more so than it seems. Buy the best quality metal for this that you can—you may have all you need already waiting in your jewelry box (along with a variety of pendants). You can buy unfinished chain from jewelry-making catalogs for less cost than finished ones. You're going to cut it to your chosen pendulum length anyway. Real silver and gold carry energy far more optimally than pot metals, and lower-grade silver is inexpensive. In choosing a chain for your pendulum, you will find that the very cheapest ones reduce the usefulness of your pendulum because they just don't carry the energy. Try the chain before you buy it.

You can hold a chain in the store, and even without a weight on the end, try using it for a pendulum. Or hang something on the end, a key or whatever might be available. It won't work as well as it will once the pendant is attached, but if you compare a couple of kinds of chain, you will definitely see the difference and know which to buy. If you are making your own pendulums, you need to use chain that is made with links. Snake-type chains can't be cut into lengths and there's nothing to hook the jump ring or head pin loop through. It is best to avoid using the thinnest and finest gauge of chain for pendulum making since it tends to knot up. Use something of medium weight.

You can also use a bracelet chain, attaching your bead and pendulum weight at each end. The length will probably be right, without your needing to cut it with your rosary pliers. A bracelet is usually about seven inches long, an ankle bracelet a bit longer. Either of these can be made into pendulums. You may not need a chain made with links for this, as you will attach your weight and bead to the rings that are already on either end. You can use the clasp on one end to hook the pendant to the chain, and use the jump ring at the other end to connect the head pin loop on your holding bead.

If you get very interested in jewelry making, you might wish to learn wire wrapping. A wire-wrapped gemstone or crystal makes a lovely, if sometimes slightly fragile, pendulum. There are many books on beadwork, bead stringing, wire wrapping, silverwork, and most other kinds of jewelry making and crafts. Bead stores, craft shops, lapidaries, and even community colleges offer how-to classes. My interest in making pendulums has extended into making gemstone bead necklaces, bracelets, ankle bracelets, earrings, and other items. My Goddess Brede likes to decorate backpacks with beads, jewelry, embroidery, and bells. Pendulum making can take you further into other crafts.

One kind of pendulum end to take note of is the Mermet pendulum, named for the French dowser who designed it. This pendulum is more familiar than it sounds, being simply a brass or other metal, or sometimes wood, pendulum or pendant that screws open to reveal a small cylindrical space inside. These are also called "witness pendulums." They were originally used by dowsers to hold a tiny sample of whatever the pendulum was being used to look for. If a dowser was looking for water, for example, she would put a few drops of water into the container part of the tool. If she was looking for a person, she might put a strand of the person's hair inside. The idea was to tune the pendulum to what it was seeking.

Mermet pendulums can still be used in this way, but you can also put other items inside them. Place a few grains of salt or sage inside to keep the pendulum clear, as these materials are purifiers. Change the salt or herbs frequently. You can also put a tiny crystal or gemstone inside; it adds to the weight and the sensitivity of the pendulum. I find heavier (but not overly large or heavy) pendulums more effective to use than lighter ones. The spaces inside these pendulums are very small, and not a lot goes in.

If you have access to water from the Chalice Well of Glastonbury, England, put a few drops inside your Mermet pendulum. This is a very potent Goddess energy that will amplify all psychic work. Drinking water from the Chalice Well is also wonderful if you have the opportunity to find it fresh or preserved as an essence. The Chalice Well is a branch of this planet's Well of Life and Light and a channel for the planetary life force. Its water is all healing, psychic opening, and a means of connecting deeply with Goddess energy. Used on your altar, especially when dedicating your pendulums (or yourself), this water is extremely sacred.

If you carry your pendulums with you, they need to be in a protective pouch of some type. You can make pouches or buy them, but they are almost too cheaply purchased to be worth the work of making them. The pendulum will stay clear longer and therefore work better if it is not left loose in a pocket or purse, or left sitting out exposed. You will also be less likely to lose it. Silk is an especially good energy protector and insulator, so you may want to use a silk drawstring pouch. It only has to be two or three inches long. I personally find drawstring closures a nuisance and prefer a pouch that closes with a snap or a zipper. My pendulums are in and out of my pocket a thousand times a day.

One possibility for a pendulum pouch is the small type of hard case used to hold a lipstick tube. Remove the mirror from the inside; with the bouncing of the pendulum against it in your pocket, it will only break. I like to tape an address label on the inside of the lid where the mirror was. Occasionally pendulums get lost, and sometimes they actually come back. These little containers are available in many stores and cost only a couple of dollars.

A small change purse also works well for a pendulum pouch. Finding them small enough can be a challenge, but they turn up sometimes in unexpected places, and they cost very little. They can be of leather, cloth, or even plastic. The mojo bag you wear around your neck is a possibility, too. You might wrap the pendulum inside it, or in any other kind of pouch, in a scrap of silk. A few grains of salt or sage in the pouch can also help to keep your pendulums energetically cleared for as long as possible. When your pendulum is not with you, it should be on your altar and in salt or under a pyramid to clear it.

If pendulum making seems like a lot of work, you can buy ready-made pendulums in stores. New Age stores are especially good sources, as are New Age catalogs. Women's bookstores often carry pendulums, as do lapidary stores, jewelry-making catalogs, some gift catalogs, and many bead stores. In this case, someone else has done the designing and choosing of materials and all the work for you. You will pay considerably more than you would if you made the pendulum yourself, often as much as thirty or thirty-five dollars for a good quality pendulum with silver findings. However, the pendulum you buy may be beautiful enough to be worth the extra cost.

There are things to look for when buying a pendulum. All the choices you made while experimenting with various types and materials of pendulums will come into play here, just as if you were designing your own pendulum. In this case, you will have to find your requirements ready-made. You may wish to make simple alterations, such as shortening the chain. Most store-bought pendulums come with a foot-long chain, too long to be comfortable for most users.

I also find that most pendulums in stores are overly large, too large to carry comfortably in a pocket or to use easily. A friend once made me several pendulums. They had wire-wrapped tumbled crystals on both ends that were nearly as large as golf balls and a foot of heavy-gauge silver chain in between. The pendant stones did not have pointed ends but were almost spherical. With both ends the same size (badly oversized) and in the wrong shape, the "pendulum" was heavy, unbalanced, and unwieldy. It was so heavy that it barely registered responses and couldn't be used. The stones were beautiful but more suited to use singly on necklaces (and probably too heavy for those) than as pendulums. The woman who made them for me meant well, but she obviously had never used pendulums herself. Many of the pendulums sold in stores have similar problems; they are too big, too heavy, too long, unbalanced, and wrongly shaped.

When looking for a pendulum in a store, first notice how it looks. Is it attractive and are you attracted to it? Don't buy a pendulum simply because you need one and it's the only one available. You can always make do with a string and paperclip until you find the right tool. If it has gemstones on it, do the energies of the stones complement each other, or do they clash? This is something you can sense as much as estimate rationally. If the colors clash, you can assume the energies do. A lapis lazuli pendulum doesn't look good with a bloodstone bead on top, and the energies won't work well together. I would also avoid a pendulum made from plastic beads—though I make these sometimes to give to children.

Look at the pendulum's findings and metal. Is the chain of nice quality? If it's too long, you can shorten it, but often store pendulums come with chains that break the first time you tug on them. You'll have to replace the chain if you buy it, probably sooner than later. Are the pendant, bead top, and mountings well made, and if there are gemstones, are they of reasonable quality for the price? Is there a bead at the end or just bare chain? Does this matter to you?

Pick up the pendulum and try working with it. Very often you will have to clear the energy and dedicate the pendulum, asking your Goddess or guide to work through it before it will work for you at all. A pendulum that doesn't feel right in the store might never work properly, but it will usually be fine once it's been cleared. You can use a pendulum you already have to ask if you should buy the new one you're considering. Hold the new one in your other hand, or touch it while you ask, and obey your guidance on the matter. If your current pendulum says "no," leave the new one in the store. If your current pendulum says "yes," you may bring the new one home.

Whether you make or buy your pendulums, you are now ready to prepare your tools for use. The next chapters discuss cleansing and dedicating your pendulums. If it seems to be taking a long time to reach the instructions for pendulum use, you will find that these preliminary preparations are extremely important groundwork and highly worthwhile. However, if you wish to read ahead to chapter six, on how to use a pendulum, you may do so at any time.

CLEANSING

What is it that makes a pendulum a psychic tool and not just an ordinary weight on a string? What turns common objects, a pendant, bead, and piece of necklace chain, into a device for communication with higher information sources than you can otherwise consciously access? It is the pendulum's ability to transmit psychic energy, information from a Goddess, angel, archangel, member of the Lords of Karma, or other high-level Be-ing of the Light. There are two important requirements that make this transmission possible: one is purification and the other is dedication. Purification, or cleansing, is the subject of this chapter, and we will discuss dedication in the next.

In order for psychic energy transmission to take place, the tool used to transmit it has to be made and kept absolutely energetically cleared. A pendulum must be an instrument of clear communication, receiving undistorted information. Clearing, or cleansing, means that there are no negative or interfering energies to block, cut, or distort the transmission, or to prevent a Light-being from being able to safely transmit her response through the tool. Likewise, since you are the means of operating the pendulum and the receiver of the energy/information, you must be dedicated to the Light (see chapter four) to be kept purified as well. This is necessary because your questions must be transmitted clearly and without distortion to the Goddess or other Light-being who is running the pendulum for you, and she must be able to clearly respond.

Your transmission of questions to the Light-being is by thought—you phrase the question in your mind. The responses are transmitted through your pendulum, and it is the energy of the answer moving through your unconscious thoughts that causes the pendulum to swing. All psychic ability, all creativity, and all Creation of every kind originate in thought, which is then transmitted into manifestation. It is the primal energy from which all is made, from which the Light/Goddess/Source creates all of life and all worlds. Thought is Creation itself. The power of thought transmission is the source of communication of all kinds, including communication using a pendulum. Clear thought means clear communication.

As all-powerful as it is, thought is a fragile energy. It can be deflected, misdirected, distorted, weakened, diverted, interfered with, and miscommunicated in any variety of ways. If you have ever meditated, you know how hard it is to clear your thoughts; if you have ever done psychic healing or visualization, you know how hard it is to focus and direct your thoughts clearly and without distraction. A pendulum is a tool for the reception of thought energy, and it must be kept cleared to prevent the energy and thought from going astray or from being stopped altogether, from being misdirected or incorrectly received.

All psychic ability is the ability to direct and focus thought, and pendulum use is a psychic ability. When you use a pendulum, you are asking a Be-ing of the Light to transmit a thought response to you that you perceive as the movement of the pendulum. It is the influence of the Light-being's thought upon your subconscious mind that creates the neuromuscular effect that makes the pendulum move. The Goddess's (or other communicator's) thought influencing your thought moves your hand, generating an involuntary movement of your hand and fingers, which makes the pendulum swing in a "yes" or "no" response. The Be-ing of the Light that offers you the answers derives them from the planetary Collective Consciousness; all minds are one mind, all thought is one thought, and all information is available to everyone. This is what makes Light-beings seem so all-knowing; they have access to the Collective Consciousness that we in body do not.

A pendulum is therefore a means of receiving information from the Collective Consciousness by way of a Light-being who finds the information you request and who then transmits it in a way that you can understand. All of this happens nearly instantaneously. She transmits it through your subconscious thought processes, to create the involuntary neuromuscular response that swings the pendulum. For the thought energy to transmit accurately and communicate as an understandable message, every stage of the process must be kept flowing without interference. Your thoughts must be kept clear, and your pendulum must be kept clear as well.

You have already seen how some pendulum-making materials transmit energy more optimally than others, and even how some materials don't transmit energy at all. Finding and using materials that transmit energy well is a significant part of creating optimal communication. Cleansing your pendulums and keeping them cleansed are the next essential steps if communication is to flow and the information you receive is to be useful and accurate.

Purification does not mean that you or your pendulum is "dirty"; this is an entirely different kind of "cleanliness." Have you ever received an electric shock in winter from walking across a wool carpet? It feels as if your feet are dragging against something unseen and clingy, and as soon as you touch something with your hand, you feel and see the spark. This is similar to what happens to a pendulum that needs clearing. The energy moving through it becomes full of static and sticky. The fragile transmission of thought is broken up, reduced, or destroyed in moving through such static. The drag and cling of the interfering energy causes the pendulum to move erratically, like being unable to walk smoothly across the carpet. Your pendulum is no longer accurate in its responses, as the information transmitted to and through you by the Light-being running it is deflected.

Another example is of radio or telephone transmission. Sometimes in a thunderstorm or sunspot cycle, radio transmission fails and the station goes off the air for a while. Sometimes the reception you receive is filled with static to the point where you can't understand what's being broadcast. Two stations may even overlap and seem to talk on top of each other. In this case, the thunder and lightning (or solar activity) are competing and interfering with the energy of the electronic transmitter. In the same way, competing energies interfere with a pendulum's ability to transmit information accurately or at all. These competing thoughts, or psychic energies, may be finer and less simple to perceive than the lightning storm.

It is easy to tell when your pendulum needs to be cleared. The most obvious indication is when it won't swing at all, when it swings erratically in an unusual way, or when the responses you receive are obviously false. For example, instead of receiving clear "yes" and "no" responses, your pendulum just spins in a circle or doesn't move. When you ask it a question with an obvious answer to test it, you get a wrong answer or series of wrong answers. You might ask the pendulum, "Is my name Jane?" when you know your name is not Jane. If the pendulum insists that your name *is* Jane, something is definitely wrong. An entity that is not of the Light may have taken over the pendulum when this happens, but usually only purification is needed.

Another way to tell when your pendulum needs cleansing is when the swing is no longer firm and clear, but sloppy and slow. It may seem apathetic or halfhearted, or the swing may seem so indecisive that you can't distinguish a "yes" from a "no." Sometimes the answers seem to come too slowly, both in how long it takes the pendulum to start to respond and in how fast and surely it swings when it does respond. Sometimes the pendulum just doesn't feel right to hold and use, something feels "off." A sluggish pendulum always needs clearing. I can almost tell when I pick a pendulum up if it's clear; the weight and heft of a cleansed pendulum feels straight and solid.

An uncleared pendulum does not transmit accurate information. You can't trust the responses you receive; some are correct and some are not, and it may be impossible to tell which are which. A pendulum reacting in this way is of no use and is not to be depended upon. A pendulum in need of purification may also swing wildly out of your hand and fall on the floor or ground, sometimes even to shatter. It almost feels as if something (or someone) has pulled it away from you, which is probably the case. This drastic reaction only happens when the pendulum is in need of clearing so badly, and you persist in using it that way for so long, that the Goddess or Light-being running it has to do something immediate to get your attention. Sometimes the shock of the fall actually clears it.

Pendulums made with crystals require purifying more often than wood pendants or those made of brass or other kinds of metal. Better quality metals, gemstones, and other materials require cleansing less often than lower quality metals, materials, and gems. Pendulums made with plastics need frequent clearing and are difficult to cleanse at all. They can't be used for very long at a time. Of natural materials that need the most clearing the most often, quartz crystal comes first, and other types of gemstones follow. Hematite seems to need clearing less often than most other colored gemstone pendants and beads. If you make your pendulums with it, however, make sure to use natural hematite and not the synthetic (hemalyke) imitations.

Your pendulum will always need to be cleared when you buy it and first bring it home. Part of what needs cleansing is the energies of many people handling pendulums, which always happens in stores. This is not to say that there is anything wrong or bad about the people, only that the confusion of mixed energies interferes with accurate pendulum use. Your own energies need to be cleared from your pendulums too, and that is a part of why they need repeated purification. Human energy has vibration, and that vibration and mix of vibrations build up on any transmitting instrument, like the static did on the wool rug. The first clearing often takes the longest, and it is tempting to skip it so you can play with your new purchase. This is the wrong thing to do, however, and a little patience now will pay off later.

Homemade pendulums also need cleansing when you first make them. I always clear the materials—the pendants, chain, and bead—before I make the pendulum, and then clear the finished tool again as soon as I complete it. New pendulums (and other psychic tools) take some time to harmonize with your energy, to become "broken in." I also find that old pendulums, those I've used for a long time, can become harder and harder to clear until finally they can't be cleared at all and have to be replaced. How long this takes varies with how much and how often you use a pendulum, how frequently you purify it, and whether you consistently keep it purified enough.

One way to know whether your pendulum is in need of cleansing is to ask the Light-being or Goddess who is running it for you. I pose this question frequently while doing pendulum work, and I take out a different pendulum as soon as I'm told that I need to. I rarely use a pendulum for more than a couple of hours, and for less time if I'm working with it intensively or constantly, before setting it aside to clear and taking out a different one. If the work you do with the pendulum is important to you, it deserves to be done well and with optimal accuracy, and this requires that your pendulums always be energetically cleared.

Occasionally an entity that is not of the Light can take over a pendulum. These can be discarnate spirits, negative elementals, attachments, or a variety of other nasties. You need to be able to recognize when this happens and what to do about it. This is when your pendulum will move in a small, fast, tight spin, round and round and round, and keep on doing it. Sometimes its responses will all be "no," no matter what you ask, and occasionally all of its responses will be "yes." While this is happening, you may have the impression that you are being laughed at in a jeering way and that something is really enjoying interfering with you—which it probably is. Occasionally you will get a visual of the entity, which may or may not be in human form.

Your response to this is to ask the pendulum, "Are you of the Light?" If it isn't, the spin will continue or worsen, you may hear or sense the nasty laugh, the pendulum may swing to communicate "no," or it may suddenly go limp as the entity lets go of it and leaves. Make a very strong mental command, "Leave now and don't come back." Ask for help from Archangel Michael or any other Protector of the Light, and also make sure that the entity leaves your home—permanently. Don't be afraid to ask that it be destroyed. Put the pendulum in a dish of dry salt for at least a week, away from your other pendulums and not on your altar. After the week, rededicate it. Take a different, cleared pendulum and ask if the entity is gone and if the pendulum is safe to use. If the answer is "no," throw the pendulum away, taking it out of your house and putting it into the garbage outdoors. When the tool has been a favorite one or was expensive, this is hard to do, but it's necessary for your safety and that of the Goddess, guide, or Light-being who runs pendulums for you. Don't look back. Something better will come to take its place.

Sometimes in situations like this, the entity is gone and the pendulum is cleansed, but it just doesn't seem to work anymore. You put it back for more clearing and more clearing, but it never feels right again. After a while, it seems obvious that the situation won't change, and you finally throw the tool away. What happened? Pendulums are made with gemstones and metals, and each of these has a life force, a spark of life and Light that animates it (even when it is non-animate by our definitions and has no ability to move). Metals have elementals, and crystals have devas in them. They are sparks of the Collective Consciousness of elements and crystals, and though not alive in the way that we are, they still are living Be-ings. Since they have life, they can also die—which in this case means that the spark of life in them returns to the Collective. Once that bit of life spark has left your pendulum, for all practical purposes the pendulum is dead. Though there is no danger to you in this situation, there is also nothing you can do about it. Discard the pendulum and make a new one.

There are a variety of ways to clear and purify pendulums. Probably the most useful of the cleansing methods is to bury your pendulums (you can usually do several at once) in a small container of dry sea salt and leave them there at least overnight. For a brand-new pendulum being purified for the first time, cover it in salt for three days to a week. The container can be glass or ceramic, or even a small cardboard jewelry box or woven basket. It should not be plastic or made of any metal other than stainless steel. Throw away the salt after each use; you will only need a few teaspoons to cover the pendulums.

Sea salt is better than table salt, because table salt contains chemicals, aluminum, and anti-caking agents that sea salt does not. If you have only table salt, however, you can use it. Sea salt is available in bulk at most health food stores; it costs about fifty cents a pound. If you buy it packaged, it is more expensive, about three dollars for a pound box, but again, you are using very little of it and a box will last for many months. Kosher salt can be used as well, but avoid sidewalk salt as it is filled with dirt and impurities—you want a salt that is food grade.

If you are cleansing a number of items at once, or if you simply prefer it, you can use salt water instead of dry salt. I use about a quarter cup of sea salt to about a pint of water. This is an extremely strong salt solution, but the purpose is cleansing, and this solution clears the items in the bowl very quickly, usually within an hour. (Ask whatever pendulum you are using at the time if the clearing is done and if you can now take the items from the bowl.) Once you finish, pour the bowl of water and salt down the sink drain—never reuse salt or salt water that has been used for cleansing. Salt can be used to clear things other than pendulums—gemstones and crystals of every kind (except "stones" like hanksite or halite that will dissolve in water), gemstone jewelry, ritual objects, pendulum or jewelry-making materials (pendants, beads, chain, and so forth).

If you are fortunate enough to reside near living salt water—the ocean—you have a whole other way of cleansing pendulums with salt. Go to the beach, taking with you the items you need to clear and a bucket or container to put water in. You can fill the bucket with water from the sea (it can be plastic, as there is less salt in seawater than in the above cleansing solution), place your objects to be cleared in it, then sit and enjoy the beach. The combination of sun and seawater leaves pendulums, crystals, gemstones, and jewelry feeling wonderful. It takes about an hour. If you wish to clear your stones and pendulums directly by taking them into the ocean with you, place them in a net lingerie bag to make sure the waves don't wash them away.

When your pendulum says that everything in the bucket is cleared, take the items out and spread them on a towel to dry and absorb the sunlight. If your pendulums or jewelry contain the following stones, however, don't put them in the sun, for they will fade: rose quartz, amethyst, kunzite, morganite, fluorite, or any other pink, blue, or purple crystalline gemstones.

Though it is probably the best cleansing medium, using salt has a couple of drawbacks. If the pendulums or other items you place in it are silver, the silver will tarnish. You can polish them again, but it's an extra task requiring a silver-polishing cloth or liquid. If you clear strung necklaces (beads strung on wire or cord), the salt will deteriorate the stringing material—not immediately or the first time, but fairly quickly. In this case, make sure to rinse the necklace off thoroughly in cold water when you take it from the salt solution. Using dry salt lessens this deterioration, but dust off the loose salt thoroughly once the cleansing is finished. Some fragile types of jewelry, made of pot metals or put together by gluing, can be damaged by salt water.

An excellent alternative to salt is placing your pendulums under a pyramid for clearing. The shape of a pyramid itself is the medium by which the purification occurs. A number of books have been written on pyramids and their mysteries. Why they work is mostly unknown, but when the proportions are correct they work very well. With the proper geometry, a pyramid can be made of anything, even cardboard. They can be of any size, from a couple of inches on each side to giant ones that fill a room. A pyramid can be open sided—made of strips or tubes of copper, plastic, or glass to delineate the shape—or closed so that you open one side to place the objects within. Some of them can be very beautiful. Align one side of the pyramid to due north to make it work.

Pyramids can be bought at New Age, gift, museum, planetarium, and science center shops. The pamphlets that come with pyramids are fascinating and will give you many ideas for other uses. Gemstone and lapidary stores often carry pyramids, because they are a good means of crystal and gemstone clearing. Look on the Internet. Prices start at about ten dollars for a small pyramid. Try to find a larger pyramid if you can, about a foot on each side is excellent. You will find so many uses for it, so many things to clear in your pyramid, that a small one won't be enough. I have two larger ones in use at all times, and they are always filled.

Pyramids clear pendulums and gemstones more slowly than dry or wet sea salt does. If you place your pendulums under a pyramid to clear, expect it to take about three days before the cleansing is complete. I use a pyramid most of the time for my pendulums (and place my gemstone jewelry in one at night as well). When a pendulum is very overloaded, however, or has a negative entity in it, or when I first bring a new one home from a store, I prefer using the very strong sea salt solution described above. If you depend on a pyramid primarily for clearing your pendulums, you will need a lot of pendulums. Once you learn to depend on this method of psychic communication, you will use it frequently, even constantly. With the longer time pyramids take for clearing, you will need to keep rotating your pendulums under the pyramid.

There are still more methods of purification and cleansing to choose from. Pendulums can be placed in the sun, at the beach or anywhere in nature, to clear them. They need to be in direct sunlight, not behind a window, for best results. Remember that some colors of gemstones fade in sunlight. Moonlight clears pendulums also, though less quickly than the sun. Place them outdoors overnight on Full or New Moons. If you have a tree in your yard, hang your pendulums from a low branch and leave them there for several hours to clear. (Occasionally a pack-rat bird, like a blackbird or crow, or a curious squirrel will carry these away.) Put them on the ground for the Earth to cleanse and purify them. Put them outdoors in a rainstorm to clear, especially if there is thunder and lightning. Make sure they are contained, so they can't wash away.

Indoors or out, running water is another means of pendulum cleansing. Water in nature is always more potent and alive than tap water, but tap water will do in a pinch. The ocean is the best outdoor source of water; running freshwater is second best. If you can hold your pendulums in a waterfall or fountain, they will clear beautifully, and you will like how they feel. Hold on tight, and don't let the water wash them away. Any water you use should be clean water. Indoors, hold your pendulum, point down, under the running faucet. Always use cold water as hot can shatter some gemstones. Keep your pendulum in the water until your guidance or intuition tells you that it's cleansed. This is a method to use when no stronger purification is available; if your pendulum is in heavy use, running water won't clear it enough. Repeat the under-the-tap clearing as often as you need to.

A variety of herbs can be used for purification. Sage and cedar are traditional Native American cleansing herbs. Place your pendulums in a bowl with a handful of dry sage for clearing. Rose petals are a lovely way to clear pendulums but are probably not strong enough for heavy-duty use when your pendulums are really overloaded. Other dry herbs you can use include frankincense, myrrh, and mugwort. Dragon's blood (a plant resin) is quite strong, but can be difficult to find. To purchase cleansing herbs, try botanicas and herb, Native American, New Age, and sometimes health food stores.

Clearing in dry herbs can take a long time, often as long as several days, but if you burn the herbs as incense and draw your pendulums through the smoke, they clear quite quickly. The herbs can be placed on a lit charcoal block for burning or can be purchased as incense sticks or cones. Sage and cedar come as bundled smudge sticks, and some purification herbs like dragon's blood come in powdered form.

Incense sticks are the easiest to use. They are easily available in many kinds of stores, and they are inexpensive. Make sure you are buying natural incense, rather than synthetic scents—don't buy from supermarkets but from New Age stores. Along with individual herbs, New Age stores will carry incense combinations of many types especially for purification purposes. Nag Champa incense is a favorite, as is Morning Star. I use a commercially prepared combination incense stick of dragon's blood and white sage that is very powerful. When you use these to clear your pendulums, the smoke is also clearing the room. Take the incense through all your rooms at least once a month to purify your home.

To use smoke for pendulum cleansing, light the end of the incense stick with a match, let it burn for a moment, and then blow out the flame. Stand the smoking stick in an incense burner or small container of rice or sand. You can also hold it by the end if you wish. Take a pendulum and place it in the smoke that rises from the incense. Hold it in the smoke and ask the Goddess or Be-ing running the pendulum to tell you when it is fully cleared. You will see the pendulum swinging "no" in the smoke; when it is cleared, the swing changes to "yes." Put the pendulum down and repeat the process with the next one, and so on, until all of your pendulums are purified and clear.

Some flower essences can be used for pendulum purification. I found a "Crystal Clearing Combination" in a New Age store years ago that is wonderful. I put a few drops in a pint sprayer bottle filled with water and the spray clears everything I use it on—pendulums, crystals and gemstones, jewelry, everything on my altar, and the altar itself. The one-ounce dropper bottle has lasted for years, but unfortunately the brand is no longer available. I make a Detox Essence of my own from yellow allemande flowers that clears very well. Bach Crab Apple Flower essence also clears pendulums. Where essences are available, use your pendulum to help you find one that will work.

Every time I pick up a pendulum from cleansing in sea salt, remove one from the pyramid I keep them under, or take one from its pouch to use, I ask the Light-being running pendulums for me, "Is this tool absolutely energetically cleared?" If it is not, I put it back for more purification. I always start out with a pendulum that is absolutely energetically cleared. While using the pendulum, I frequently ask, "Is this pendulum clear enough to keep using for now?" The accuracy and value of your pendulum-derived information depends upon it being kept as absolutely energetically cleared as possible at all times.

While it takes a bit of thought and effort to keep your pendulums in this purified state, the effort is worthwhile, and it is truly necessary. Of the many reasons why pendulums can be inaccurate and undependable, not being maintained in an energetically cleared state is the primary one. For many users, pendulums have the reputation of being limited in the kind and quality of information you can use them for. My friends tell me, "Pendulums lie," or "They'll say anything you want them to say." This is true when they are used improperly, when they are not dedicated, and especially when they are not kept absolutely energetically cleared. The purpose of this book is to teach you to use pendulums more accurately and for more uses than you have ever known before. Cleansing is essential; it is the key to these advanced uses and to your success and accuracy in employing them.

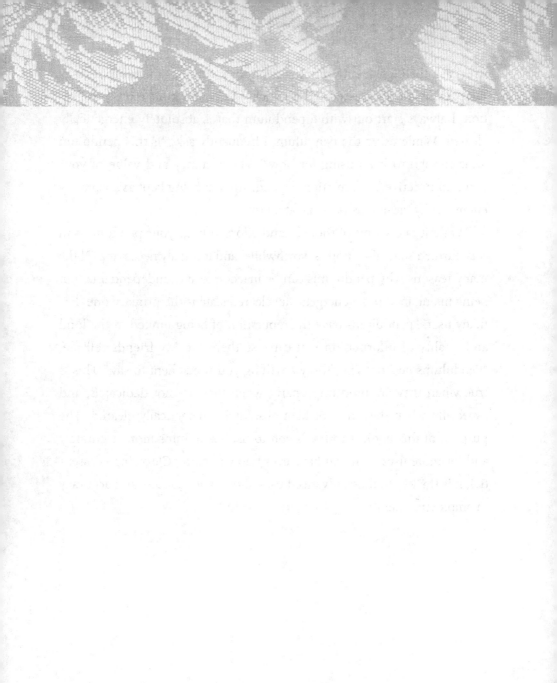

DEDICATION TO THE LIGHT

The previous chapter discussed cleansing and purification, and this must be done before a pendulum or person is dedicated to the Light. Dedication is a necessary step if you want your pendulums to be more than toys, since the Light cannot work directly through an undedicated tool—or even an undedicated person. Only when dedicated can the pendulum become a serious healing or psychic tool. When you do a dedication, you are stating in unequivocal terms that only the Light is welcome. You are inviting the Light to work through you, and you are renouncing all that is not the Light, all that is negative, manipulative, or evil. Doing this is a sacred act, not to be taken without thought and an understanding of what you are doing. If it is only your pendulum you are dedicating, it is of less consequence than if you are also dedicating yourself.

Your actions have consequences and so does your life. Your thoughts have consequences as well—possibly primary consequences considering that thought is the raw material of all creation and action. Women especially have taken the hard road in learning this fact, and it's important that we learn it now. We have been kept secondary and dependent for many thousands of years. In the herstory of our Creation, this is a reversal of what was in the beginning and of what was meant to be. Women are the bearers of new life and were the originators of all of life. God, in the concept's first intention, was female. We were invaded and taken over, again and again, and Earth became a patriarchy. It was not a just patriarchy that valued all of life, but a destructive and evil one that destroyed it and destroyed life's originators. Women were reduced to servants. We lost the knowledge of who we are and where we came from, and we lost our freedom.

Men were also reduced, enslaved, and duped, but they came out on top. Where women were denied the independence and consequence of their actions and even of their thoughts, men's actions and thoughts became distorted and skewed. In the plan of our Creation, men served the Goddess and the Light; they revered the female and were women's partners and protectors. On Earth, and in our herstory before Earth, men became oppressors instead of protectors. Men's actions became independent, but men were still lacking in the awareness and understanding of consequence. To give an example, in allowing our planet to be exploited and polluted, the patriarchal system forgets that it is destroying its own means of sustenance and survival. In oppressing women, men forget that they are oppressing their mothers and themselves. Men also need to learn that their actions have consequences and to respect the consequences before they act.

Some Native American teaching requires the examination of every action, before it is committed, to determine its consequences to the next seven generations. This is the place to start. This understanding of what you do, and that what you do extends far into the future for yourself and others, is vital if the Earth is to survive. Considering the consequences is not only important for the larger actions but for every action, no matter how small. Women need to learn that what they do can change the world. Men need to be aware that what they do has changed and is changing the world, and not always in positive ways. Everyone needs to be aware of the consequences of their every act, and of how each act affects them, affects all they love, affects the generations to come, and affects the planet.

For more information on where we really came from, the herstory that has been lost and kept from our knowledge, see my books *Essential Energy Balancing II: Healing the Goddess* and the forthcoming *Essential Energy Balancing III: Living with the Goddess.* People were created as

Light-beings, and our evolutionary job is to return to that status. Understanding that you are a Creator, and making sure that what you create is only of the Light, is an absolutely necessary first step. This is true no matter how small what you are creating seems to be. Your thoughts, actions, creations, and life all have consequences, and those consequences must be only of the Light.

Why does there need to be so much emphasis on this? Isn't it enough to do what you know is right and to do the best you can? Yes and no. It is certainly important to do good things and to live your life in that manner. It is also not enough; there is real evil in the world. Despite how fundamentalist that sounds, and I am not a fundamentalist, it is so. Listen to a newscast any day for any number of examples of evil. Everyone has experienced it individually as well. No life is untouched by it. There are countless wrongs happening every day, in every moment of our lives and in every moment of all of life. You may realize this but say, "There's nothing I can do about it; it's just how things are. Who am I to change the world?" You are the only thing that *can* change the world.

Change starts with you. Each individual act and thought that serves the Light serves you and changes you. And when many people understand this and act accordingly, serving the Light and making change in themselves in every small way that they can, the balance shifts. We then reach a point of critical mass, and that's where the world begins to change. Critical mass is reached when enough individuals have made a change in their awareness, hopefully for the better, and their change becomes part of the Collective Consciousness. It doesn't take a great many people to cause this shift to occur, far less than most of us believe. What you do has consequences, and all change—for all of life—begins with you.

So where do we start? By dedicating yourself to the Light. How to do this is discussed below. Performing this dedication has to be a considered act, however, and I want to talk about what it means before you do it. Even though you have spent your life until now doing the best you can, with every intention of doing good, a great deal of your life will change when you make the dedication. The act is a statement that you are ready to be a part of the solution and no longer a part of the problems facing life on Earth. You won't be expected to change everything and everyone, however, but only to change yourself. Dedication initiates great internal change. When the Light comes in, all that is not the Light leaves. You may find yourself becoming a very different person—starting a new career, finding a new place to live, choosing a new relationship or way of life, thinking and feeling differently. Whatever is not working in your life will end, whether that be a bad marriage or a bad habit.

I watch this happen repeatedly with my Reiki students, and receiving Reiki, with the intent to serve, is its own dedication to the Light. By the time a year has passed after the teaching weekend, I almost don't recognize some of my students. They have changed that much. They tell me that it's been a hard year, a rough ride. When I ask them if they regret it, no one does. When I ask them whether they are happy now, the answer is always yes, or that they are approaching happiness. This is what happens when you dedicate yourself to the Light. You will also find that every kind of blessing that seemed out of reach before becomes available now. You will have a new and vastly better life.

Dedication to the Light is a spiritual act, not a religious one. It is in accordance with all religions and all religious thought. Anyone can do this. If you feel the need to do it in a church or other place sacred to religion, you are welcome to do so. You can do it out in nature, and you can do it at home. It is a sacred, serious act and needs to be recognized as such and done in a respectful way. Don't try it in a traffic jam; find a quiet place where you can spend some time beforehand thinking about why you choose to do it. Spend some quiet time afterward waiting for impressions that will come; such impressions, thoughts, and information can be extremely important to you. How all this applies to using pendulums comes later.

In its simplest form, here is how to dedicate yourself. First choose a quiet place where you will not be disturbed, indoors or in nature. Sit quietly and still for a few minutes and calm yourself inside. Light a candle, which represents the Light and brings angels and Light-beings to you. The candle puts the Light on notice that you are doing spiritual work. You may smudge yourself with incense smoke for cleansing, as you did your pendulums. Then make a simple statement: "I dedicate myself and my life, and all my lifetimes and between them, to the Light." Repeat it two more times. Then sit quietly for a while and see what comes. If there is a particular Light-being you wish to dedicate yourself to—a specific Goddess, God, angel, saint, or Lord of Karma, for example—you may now do so in the same way. Add to the statement you made above saying, "I also dedicate myself to Isis," or whomever of the Light you have a special affinity for.

If you already have an altar, it's the obvious place to make your dedication; if not, you can easily make yourself an altar if you wish to. An altar is simply a representation of the four elements (Earth, Air, Fire, and Water), and the fifth element of Spirit or Ether. Represent these by a crystal for Earth, incense for Air, a candle for Fire, a seashell or bowl of salt water for Water. Place these in a circle on a scarf or pretty piece of cloth. Light your incense and candle. For Spirit, an object to place in the center is anything that represents divinity. Use a Goddess image, a picture of an angel or an ancestor, a sacred symbol, or whatever else may be important to you. If you choose a religious symbol, use something that affirms life instead of death or tragedy. Dedication to the Light is a celebration; the Light-beings that protect us and watch over us have been waiting for you to do it for a very long time. Do it with great joy.

If you wish to do your dedication as a formal Goddess or Wiccan ritual, you are also welcome to do so. Smudge with incense to purify, cast your circle, call in the Guardians of the Directions. When you are ready, make the statement: "I dedicate myself and my life, and all my lifetimes and between them, to the Light." If you have a particular Goddess you can add, "I dedicate myself to Brede [or Isis, or Freya, or whoever your Goddess may be]." Sit quietly within your circle for a while to see what impressions may come. Then open the circle, snuff your candle and incense, and you are finished.

Once you have dedicated yourself to the Light, Be-ings of the Light are able to work through you. Your dedication gives them the safety to be able to do so. The Light is not invulnerable to evil, any more than people are. Light-beings need protection, and so do you. The dedication puts out a warning to anything and everything that is not of the Light that it is unwelcome and that it will be sent away or destroyed if it tries to interfere with you. It also gives the Protectors of the Light permission to protect you and permission to defend you from anything that is not of the Light. They will not do this without your permission, as the Light will not violate your free will. Your dedication is a request for their help and is a powerful protection that you will have many occasions to be grateful for.

Now that Light-beings can work through you, they will be glad to do so. They have been waiting for the opportunity. Your psychic abilities will develop, your ability to achieve guidance will increase, you will be drawn to the means and methods you need to access the Light ever more fully in your life. And now because it is safe for them to do so, Be-ings of the Light will be able to work through your pendulum, through your subconscious (and conscious) mind and neuromuscular system, to communicate with you and give you information and guidance. You may also develop clairaudience (psychic hearing), by which you gain information through hearing it spoken. You will then hear Light-beings directly, without the intermediary of the pendulum tool. You may develop other abilities—clairvoyance, healing, and so on.

Once you have dedicated yourself and cleansed your pendulums, the next step is to dedicate them and formally ask a Be-ing of the Light to work through them. You need to state in no uncertain terms that *only* a Be-ing of the Highest Light is, or will ever be, welcome. This request will be for all of your pendulum use and pendulums at once, not only for one single pendulum. As you buy or make more pendulums, however, you will want to repeat this request with each new one when you dedicate it. Sit in front of your altar or in the quiet space you used before, this time with however many pendulums you own placed on the altar in front of you or held in your hand. Make the statement, "I dedicate this pendulum [or pendulums] to the Light, and only to the Light, and ask that a Be-ing of the Highest Light work through it always." You might also say, "I dedicate these pendulums to truth, and I ask that they always be accurate and truthful."

This is not limited to pendulums, of course, but can and should be done for every spiritual tool that you use. The items on your altar and your altar itself should all be dedicated, for example. As a writer, I've dedicated my computer and everything I do or create on it to the Light, and I have also dedicated my home and garden, pets, car, every crystal and gemstone I own, every piece of jewelry, and much, much more. I usually do this by giving them Reiki attunements while making the dedication statements above. The attunement is not enough in itself; you need to state specifically that you are dedicating the items to the Light. You can hold pendulums and small items in your hand to do this, or if what you are dedicating is too large, trace the Reiki symbols in the air over or in front of the object. If you have been trained in Reiki, you can dedicate yourself this way, by self-attunement, as well.

I did my first dedication to the Light and to my Goddess Brede at Candlemas (February 2) 1978. I repeat it every year at Candlemas and occasionally at other times. You may also wish to repeat your dedication, as well as repeat the dedication of your pendulums. When I bring home materials for pendulum making (or for making anything else), I immediately clear, attune, and dedicate them. Once I have made my pendulum from the materials, I immediately dedicate the completed tool as well, then place it under a pyramid for several days to clear again. Sometimes I dedicate it once more before its first use. I also do this for every pendulum I buy, often in the store before even trying it out. I dedicate it only to the Light at that point, so if I choose not to buy it, the tool will be

Light-dedicated for whoever takes it home, without being specifically dedicated to a Light-being that may not be the favorite of another buyer.

Now that your pendulums are dedicated, you can make contact with the Light-being who will run them. At first there will be only one Be-ing, but eventually there may be several members of the Light who will run pendulums for you—one at a time, of course. You will usually know who is there, or you can ask. They will run whichever pendulum you may be using at the time. The Light-beings are not attached to a specific pendulum, so all your pendulums should be dedicated to the Light and kept energetically cleared always for any Light-being to use. Sitting quietly, pick up a dedicated pendulum by the bead at the top, with the weight dangling free. Ask if a Be-ing of the Highest Light is willing to run your pendulums for you. Your pendulum will swing to "yes."

Ask if a Light-being is now running your pendulum. You will receive a "yes" again. Ask if that Be-ing is someone you know or have already done work with. This will probably also be "yes." Does a name come to mind? Ask if that is the name of the Light-being who is running your pendulum. It will probably be "yes" again. If the response is "no," think of other names of who it could be, and ask one by one. Sometimes the name will remain unknown for a while, but you will probably get it eventually. As long as it is a Be-ing of the Highest Light running your pendulum, whether you know his or her name or not, trust the Be-ing. As long as your pendulum is clear and your questions are clearly asked, you can usually trust the information that comes from them. Every time you pick up the pendulum to use, ask if a Be-ing of Highest Light is running it. If you know the Be-ing's name, use it and ask if he or she is there.

It needs to be said that you are to treat these Light-beings with extreme respect. Say "please" and "thank you," and thank them for working with you. Every time and with every request, you need to do this. Never speak disrespectfully, yell at Light-beings, or demand of them to do anything. If they can't or won't answer something you ask, there is always a reason for it. If they can't or won't do something you want them to do, ditto. The

Light, whether Goddess or God, angel, archangel, member of the Lords of Karma, or Divine Director, requires respect but not worship. Light-beings will not permit you to worship them. But they do expect you to work with them in a cooperative, co-creative, and polite way. It's one of the few things they ask of your relationship with them, and it is very little to ask. The other thing they ask of you, indeed insist upon, is that your work with them be only of the Light. They will not help you with or participate in anything that is not.

What does this mean? Some things are obvious. They will not allow you to do harm to yourself, to anyone else (human or nonhuman), or to the Earth. They will also not allow you to interfere with others' free will; this can cross some fine and tricky lines sometimes and be far less obvious. You will not be allowed to ask for things or information for other people, unless you request to do so and have their permission . You will not be permitted to invade others' privacy—no answers to your inquiries will be given. You will not be allowed to violate others' karma, whether you think it's for their own good or not. If you receive information for others, you are obligated to tell them what you've learned, using whatever tact may be required. If you are too embarrassed to do that, it's a good indication that these are questions you should not ask. Healers also have to learn and respect these ethics, and they come with every kind and use of psychic ability. Their violation is very serious, karmically and in every other way. Your questions with the pendulum will be mostly for yourself.

One odd aspect of these ethics is that no Light-beings will ever help you to gamble. You will not be guided in picking lottery numbers, for example, or helped to win a racing bet. I can understand this, as when I worked as a waitress I saw many women exploited by their hopes of winning millions. They studied numbers books, dream books, even fortune cookie messages, and seemed to talk of nothing else but what numbers to pick and who had recently won or lost. Waitresses make very little money, or at least these ones did. They gave away needed dollars that only went to fund the state—a state that misused lots of money and didn't need to take what little these women could earn.

Because of this awareness, I have never bought a lottery ticket. I actually seem to have reverse, or anti-psychic, ability at Bingo or gambling games. I can go through a whole game of Bingo and have nothing on my card at the end. Don't expect your pendulum or the Be-ing running it to help you pick or win at betting or numbers. Apparently it's the Light who picks these winners, notwithstanding our wants and desires.

How much can you trust the information that comes to you through a pendulum? Once you have a Be-ing of the Highest Light running it, you can trust it much more than you ever have before. This is the primary factor that makes a pendulum useful and accurate, the difference between a party game and a legitimate healing and psychic tool. This does not mean that you forgo common sense. If a response seems unlikely, or you know that it is false, take no action based on the information until you know more and know what is real and true. If the responses you receive are repeatedly unlikely, exchange your pendulum for one that you know is fully cleared.

If your responses still seem incorrect, try to find out why. First ask if a Be-ing of the Highest Light is running your pendulum. If not, tell whoever or whatever is running it to leave. Sometimes that's enough, but if the entity doesn't leave, call upon the Protectors of the Light, asking them to either take it to where it belongs or to destroy it. If it is evil, you want it destroyed, but if it is only something in the wrong place and perhaps in need of help, ask the Protectors of the Light to take care of it. Make the request something like this: "If the entity is evil, destroy it; if it's lost, take it to where it needs to go and find it the help it needs." If a negative entity has taken over your pendulum, clear the pendulum thoroughly in salt, but this may not be enough. If it still doesn't work, throw it away.

If a Be-ing of the Light running your pendulum has told you that your pendulum is not in need of cleansing, and you are still receiving implausible answers, try rephrasing your questions. If your question is not clear, your response may not be. Perhaps you are asking the wrong questions or looking at the wrong aspect of a problem. Perhaps the situation is still in flux, and until a direction is chosen, there can be no answer. Sometimes it's just not time for you to know, and your guide is not permitted to reveal the information yet. Perhaps you are asking questions you ethically should not be asking. If it is information you are not meant to have, or it violates someone's privacy, you might receive responses that are meaningless.

Occasionally, your Light-being may not know the answer. They are not in body, after all, and may not understand how things work on Earth. Use the pendulum to ask her whether or not she knows. If she doesn't, ask her if there is someone else of the Light who does know and who would be willing to tell you. That Be-ing could either run your pendulum while you need her expertise, or she can relay the information to your usual pendulum-running Goddess or angel.

In many situations, however, the information that seems unlikely is actually correct. A Goddess, God, angel, member of the Lords of Karma, or other Light-being will not deceive you and is rarely in error. There can be miscommunication, and this is more likely if you are just beginning to do pendulum work with Light-beings than if you are more experienced. Sometimes you just have to learn to trust. If you have asked the question in a different way, or a couple of different ways, and still get the same response, consider that the answer may be correct and your understanding of the situation may be incomplete or faulty.

Some people ask their Higher Self to run pendulums for them, but if you ask for a Light-being of the Highest Light, you will rarely have your Higher Self running your pendulum. Though your Higher Self has more information and a clearer perspective than you do, she is not of the *highest* Light. Likewise with spirit guides, who are only of a slightly higher level than the people in body they guide. In the request for a Be-ing of the Highest Light, we are aiming for the greatest truths we can access, going as high as we can be permitted to go for information. There are several types of Be-ings who are included in the category of "highest": angels, archangels, Goddesses and their male Twin Flames (Gods), members of the Lords of Karma (Ascended Masters), and Divine Director (to contact once you become more advanced).

Angels were created to be protectors and guides for people in body. They were created specifically for this purpose and are assigned to a particular person. You may have one or several angels assigned to you, and they may be male or female. They have the role of providing guidance, healing, and protection at once. Angels are not spirit guides. Spirit guides are people who have died and have been given the job of guiding someone that is on a level of evolution just below theirs. They know more than we do but are very much in training. Angels and archangels, however, belong to an entirely different soul group from that of people. They are of a different realm and category of the Light. The angels created for work on Earth were genetically constructed for the purpose by the archangels and our Great Mother Nada.

Archangels are the next higher level of the Angelic Realm, and their work is planetary rather than individual. If your spiritual work is in service to the planet or beyond, Archangels may be assigned to assist you. The Angelic Realm is made up of the Protectors of the Light, and there are a number of levels and types of angelic Be-ings. Archangels work on Earth and up to the beginnings of the Cosmic level. This means that their jurisdiction is the Earth, Moon, Solar System, Galaxy, and Universe. The next level above the Universe is the Cosmos, and from the Universal level and beyond, the protectors are the Elohim and some other categories of this realm. The Guardians of the Four Directions—Michael, Gabriel, Raphael, and Uriel—work close to Earth. If you need protection, you may call upon them. They may also choose to offer guidance through your pendulum. These great warriors of the Light are also some of our greatest healers. They are both male and female, many females of every realm and level of the Light are warriors and protectors.

Goddesses are the Creators and Mothers of the Light and of all of life. Wiccans say, "There is one Goddess, but She has ten thousand names." These are the Mothers of Creation known to every culture, country, and religion. They are very much beloved, and they love us as deeply as all who know them love them. Every Light-being is pure love, but the Goddesses are love personified. Many people have a Goddess that is their special favorite, and that Goddess is probably very much aware of them as well. The Goddesses are returning to Earth now for the first time in more than a thousand years. They want to be here, they have work to do for the reclaiming of this planet and of women, and they are very curious about life on Earth. If you are on the Ascension path, you may be fortunate enough to have a Goddess choose to join with you and to work through you permanently. Once that happens, your life will never be the same!

For the first time in several thousand years, the Goddesses are reuniting and rejoining with their Twin Flames. These Men of the Light—Gods, but not in the Christian sense of that word—are the twin brothers and consorts of the Goddesses. Light-beings are born in Twin Flame pairs; in the Angelic Realm these are same-sex pairs, while for Goddesses and Gods they are twins of opposite sex. There is great rejoicing that the reunion of Twin Flame pairs is able to take place at last. A very few Men of the Light will join with men in body, as the Goddesses are now joining with women. Men in body have much evolving to do before the Gods can return to Earth. These Men of the Light are quite different from men as we know them here. They have no anger or violence in their thoughts or actions, they love all women as their Mothers and Creators, and, like the Goddesses, they are Be-ings of absolute love. A few are choosing to come closer to Earth, and some may choose to run pendulums and have other interactions with people. Some of these Gods are known from mythology, but many are new. (Mythology is the remnant of our herstory; there is always something in it that is truth.)

The Lords of Karma are Ascended Masters, who have in their keeping the administration of karma to all members of all souls of the Light who incarnate in bodies on Earth. They are male and female and, like all other Light-beings, they are of every culture, race, age, and ethnic group. There are other Ascended Masters with other jobs, but only the Lords of Karma will have close contact and communication with most people. They are willing to run pendulums, and pendulums are an excellent way to work with them. Our Multi-Cosmic Great Mother Nada is the keeper and final authority of karma on Earth and in our Multi-Cosmic System, and the Lords of Karma work with and for her.

At this time of great evolutionary change, people on Earth have been granted the greatest of gifts. We have been given the means and the help to heal and release our karma simply by asking. The gift comes from Nada and is directed by the Lords of Karma for almost everyone who chooses to do the work. This divine dispensation is also the release of our greatest suffering. Once all our Earth karma is completed or released, we are no longer required to reincarnate. Understand, however, that karma comes on many levels and that clearing Earth karma is only the beginning. Beyond Earth there is the Moon, Solar System, Galaxy, Universe, Cosmos, Multi-Cosmos, Multi-Cosmic System, Multi-Verse, and Infini-Verse. An Ascended Master who is a member of the Lords of Karma has completed and released all of his or her own karma through the Cosmic level or beyond.

The final chapter of this book deals entirely with using your pendulum to work with the Lords of Karma. I have also written several books on this subject, as I consider karmic dispensation to be of vital urgency to the Earth and all people. When you begin to work with the Lords of Karma, you place yourself on the path of spiritual evolution and Ascension. If you are willing to take the initiative, there is no limit to how far you can go in healing your karma and your life. When enough people are doing this work, the law of critical mass will bring its gifts into the Collective Consciousness, where the changes will benefit everyone.

If you complete the work of releasing and healing your Earth, Moon, and Solar System karma, and begin the work at the Galactic level, you will leave the Lords of Karma behind and move on to work with Divine Director. This is the title, not the name, of a Be-ing of the Highest Light who is the administrator of karma from the Galactic through Cosmic levels. Clearing your karma this far is well within your reach if you are willing to do the work. A number of Light-beings called Presences of the Light are authorized to work with you for releasing your karma at this level. If you ask for Divine Director, the Presence who has chosen to work with you will appear—you do not choose, the Light chooses. Some of the Be-ings who do this work are Kwan Yin, Jesus, Isis, Metatron, The Shekinah, and a number of others, male and female. El Morya, who is Nada's Twin Flame, is now in charge of this position, and He may be the Be-ing who communicates with you if you reach this level.

Any of these Be-ings of the Highest Light can choose to communicate with you by pendulum. They are willing to use this tool as a means of reaching and helping more people, especially those who would not be able to communicate with them otherwise. We are in a time of very great change for the better on Earth, and many Light-beings are here to aid the shift from Dark to Light. When you use the pendulum as a means of working with these great Be-ings, you have access to a great many blessings. When you use the pendulum in this way, with absolute responsibility and integrity, you will have a tool that brings you great rewards and gifts. If you have ever been told that a pendulum is useless, you will soon learn otherwise. Respect the tool and respect the gifts of those who are choosing to make use of it to help you, to protect you, heal you, and to give you communication with the Light.

THE MEDITATIVE STATE

If your pendulum is to be accurate or to work at all, you must be able to focus your mind. Your thoughts have to be on your question, and only on your question, and they must be held steady in that focus until you receive and understand the pendulum's response. If your mind wanders, your pendulum will wander, and when pendulums don't work or give false or implausible answers, this is often the cause. Communication with the Light is thought transmission, and if the response is to be clear, your transmission of the question has to be clear. The return transmission, the information given to you by the Light-being working with you, also has to be kept completely clear, and this is done by and through your fully focused mind. Without that focus, your question cannot be transmitted and the response cannot be received without distortion.

As discussed earlier, thought transmission is a very fragile energy. The process for bringing the thoughts of the Light to our conscious access and awareness is also quite fragile. The Be-ings of the Highest Light that agree to help us in our quest for spirituality and evolution reside on a different dimension and plane of existence from ours. They are not in body as we are. And the body itself, with all its Earth consciousness and physicality, is not tuned to the dimension where the Light resides. This is not how our Creators meant for us to be, but it is how we are now. It is what we have left to us after millennia of separation from the Light, which also was not meant to happen. In our Earth incarnations, we are focused on Earth and on our lives on Earth, and we are tied to our bodies. That communication happens at all between dimensions, between Be-ings in body and those that are not in body, is a miracle.

For communication so tenuous and difficult to be given and received, the conditions have to be optimal. Yet those of us who are in body are rarely trained to establish these conditions. Our minds are the tools, and we are not taught to use them to transcend the dimensions. We are focused on our daily lives, which surround us completely. We are also immersed in a sea of noise that surrounds us and which acts as a wall of static to effectively block out transmissions that must travel by quiet or subconscious thought. Earth is a noisy place, even by our own standards, though we learn quite early to shut out the many interferences. Televisions, radios, and other media devices run constantly, and we are rarely in a quiet room except to sleep—if then. We talk and talk but rarely learn to be good listeners. Even our quiet is not quiet.

When my beloved Goddess Brede first joined with me, She found the noise of Earth almost unbearable. Her hearing is far more acute than mine, and She had never been subjected to the constant noise vibration that we who are in body live in. She couldn't shut it out as we can. I play the radio all day and through a lot of the night, and I had to turn it off. She said it hurt Her. Even in the quiet, which I found too quiet, She had frequent startle reactions that I didn't understand. When I asked Her what was frightening Her, She couldn't explain it at first. Finally, I learned that what was so auditorily painful to Her were such things as a car going by outside, or the air-conditioning and refrigerator turning on and off (which I don't even hear unless I purposely listen for them). She asked me how I could live in all of this "vibration," and I didn't understand what She meant.

I didn't know how to help Her. I offered Her "psychic earplugs" and psychically gave Her a "knob" by which to turn the volume down. It wasn't enough. Sometimes Her startle reactions, which I felt in myself but then had to discover the source of, were so bad that I would drop and break things. I entered into panic attacks that were not my own. After a couple of weeks of this, and missing the music I like so much, I had to do something. My life is quieter than most people's, but I couldn't keep it as quiet as Brede needed to be comfortable. We went to Nada, our Great Mother, and asked Her for help.

Nada talked with Brede for a while and tried to give us a solution. Brede wanted to stay with me, and I certainly wanted Her to, but we needed help. Since there were (and are) many others of the Goddesses and Gods coming to live on Earth at this time, it was an issue for all of them, for the people bringing them in, and for the Goddesses' and Gods' abilities to remain here. I had to travel in the next few days and was especially concerned that Brede would be hurt by the noise of airports and airplanes. These were always uncomfortable and draining for me and could only be much more so for Her. We talked with Nada, leaving the problem in Her hands, and the next day started our trip.

At first, Brede seemed able to handle the airport noise, though She was wary of the situation; the volume and chaos were quite uncomfortable for me too. After three weeks of keeping my life so silent, I was becoming noise sensitized as well. When we got on the plane, I warned Brede that this would be loud, and She said She was ready. As the plane started to taxi, She put Her head on my shoulder and seemed to go to sleep. "Are you alright?" I asked Her; She said She was. I could see Her and feel Her, but She didn't talk to me again until She "woke up" when we got off the plane.

Well, this was better, or seemed to be for Her, but it wasn't the best solution. She'd had to make herself the equivalent of unconscious to tolerate it. We discussed it again and talked again to Nada, who was also coming to live on Earth and would need the help for Herself too. Nada then experimented on Herself to create what was needed for everyone. Eventually, She gave Brede and the other Goddesses and Gods something She called "filters." These are apparently internal means by which they can adjust their hearing selectively. They can turn down the sound of the computer fan but still hear the birds. In my work of the last few years of bringing the Goddesses and Gods back to Earth, one thing that had to be adjusted here was the planet's own intrinsic vibration. This was probably the real source of Brede's discomfort and has hopefully been corrected now.

The same overwhelm of vibration that made Brede so uncomfortable saturates us with background noise that we don't even notice but that prevents us from hearing the finer and quieter frequencies of the Light. Where there is a babble of background noise, quieter sounds are lost, and only the louder ones are heard. While Light-beings' hearing is obviously superior and more acute than ours, the noise of Earth prevents them from hearing us as much as it prevents us from hearing them—or even more so. The answer to this is that people who want the communication have to find a way to make their minds quiet, so the transmission and reception can be heard. The Light-beings can't do this for us; they are not on Earth, and therefore it is up to us who are.

A mind made as quiet as possible is necessary for pendulum transmission and reception (and for all psychic ability) for all of the reasons above. Once made quiet, your mind must also be focused on what you wish to receive. Quiet in itself is not enough—a turned off radio doesn't give you music; you have to turn it on and tune it to a station. Many people tell me that they have no psychic abilities. When I work with them, however, I find that nearly everyone is psychic, but they have to learn to listen to what's there. They have to make their minds quiet and focused to be able to receive psychic energy. Most of us in the West are not trained to do this, and it's a skill we are sorely missing. Most of us have no idea why such skills are needed, and this in itself is unfortunate.

While it is focused attention that's needed to run a pendulum, the basic skill for learning this is *meditation*. This is the basis for every psychic ability, and every plan and process of psychic development depend upon it. Meditation is the skill of emptying your mind, making it quiet so the Light can come in. For most of us in the West, it's a difficult skill to learn, but only because we try to do it in the way that it's done in India, Tibet, or Japan. People raised in Eastern religions (Hinduism, Buddhism, Zen) and in some Native American cultures are taught the techniques of the quiet mind from a very early age. We in the West, whose minds are much busier, lives much noisier, and who rarely slow down our bodies, find meditation difficult or impossible to learn because we come to it first as adults and because it is so different from the demands of our high-tech culture.

Still, with patience, it can be learned, and many people learn it, to their total benefit. I will give you a brief description of Eastern meditation, and I suggest that you try it. Don't expect to master it on the first sitting (Westerners expect everything instantly, but life doesn't work that way). If this form of meditation interests you, practice it for twenty minutes every day, ten minutes in the morning and ten minutes before sleep at night, and over time you will become proficient. If you take this route, you will be glad you did. Your psychic abilities and ability to communicate with the Light will develop and grow in every way. Your blood pressure will also come down, your insomnia will disappear, you will find you are calmer in every aspect of your life, you will get along better with the people around you, you will live longer, and you will be healthier and happier in every way.

First, to have a quiet mind, you need to be alone and in a quiet environment. Turn off the television, radio, VCR, DVD player, and all the other noise you surround yourself with. Unplug the phones—all of them—today's cell phones are a persistent nuisance. Go into the room where your altar is and close the door. You must do this alone, as other people will only be a distraction, but if your dog or cat follows you, let them come. They can teach you everything about meditation that you need to know. If you are Wiccan and choose to cast a circle of protection for this, you are welcome to do so. Light a candle and incense. The candle is especially good as a focusing tool, and it always puts the Light on notice that you are there for them. Sit on a straight-backed chair or on the floor, whichever is the most comfortable, keeping your arms and legs uncrossed. Don't attempt a lotus position unless you are very comfortable in your body when doing it.

Sit with your back straight; pick a comfortable position and don't move around. Look steadily at the candle flame and take a few deep, slow breaths. Rock your body slowly forward and back once or twice, then from side to side, and then come back to the center. This will ground and center you, making you calm and steady, and it feels wonderful. Take all the things worrying you, everything you can't stop thinking about, and name them one by one. As you name each, imagine burning it up in the candle flame or putting it in a box to keep for later. Take whatever time you need for this. Keep your breathing slow and steady, fuller and deeper than is usual in ordinary sedentary activity. Sit still for a moment and look at the candle flame. (What you do with the candle flame, you can also do by looking into a small bowl of water. The bowl should be of a dark, solid color.)

Make yourself very still inside and out, and make the inner statement that your mind will now be very quiet. Look at the candle flame and focus your thoughts on it. You will find that you are thinking about something, that your mind is neither still nor empty. Notice what you are thinking, then let the thought drift away. With each thought that comes, and there will be lots of them, notice them, and then will them away. At first, and especially if you are new at this, the thoughts will come and come. One will leave, and the next comes. Several thoughts come at once. They will be every kind of thought, including thoughts that you will wonder why you're even thinking. Notice them and send them away. As you sit longer, the thoughts drifting in will slow. Once you are very experienced at this, they may even stop for a few moments at a time—and that is the purpose of all forms of Eastern meditation. You will feel wonderful in those moments. Buddhists call the parade of thoughts, and our typical difficulty in emptying them, the Monkey Mind.

Don't be frustrated that the thoughts keep coming and that you aren't likely to find the moment of quiet right away. It may take months of doing this for ten minutes twice a day before you experience the empty mind for the first time. And when the emptiness comes, it will come for only a moment. You will fight to regain it, but to do that you have to start the process all over again each time. Eventually you will learn to meditate. The process is the purpose here, so don't consider it a failure if your mind doesn't become quiet or hold the quiet. Do it every day, and it will get easier and easier, and the benefits to your life will grow. Even if you think that you've failed, you haven't failed at all.

This is a basic form of traditional Eastern meditation. It is well worth the time it takes to do it, and well worth making it a part of your everyday life. Though this method of meditation is optimal for the pendulum work we are doing, there are many other forms of meditation, many methods of achieving the quiet or focused mind. Meditation can be done with chants or mantras (your own personal chant), with processes such as yoga, t'ai chi, or Chi Gong, by visualization as in psychic healing, and by focused breathing techniques. It can be done by taking guided psychic journeys, by drawing energy and color in and out of your chakras, and by contemplation (similar to the pendulum meditation below). It can be done in countless other ways and teaching methods.

Try a different kind of meditation from my book *Psychic Healing with Spirit Guides and Angels*. This technique for meditating involves focusing upon the breath, which is both a Western and Eastern meditation form. Do it after you have done your ten minutes of emptying the mind or in place of the other meditation. Exhale first, then close the right nostril with your right thumb. Inhale through the left nostril slowly to the count of four. Now close the left nostril with your right index finger, and hold your breath, counting to sixteen. Lift your thumb from your right nostril and exhale to the count of eight. Repeat by leaving your index finger on the left nostril and inhaling through the right side to begin again. This is one full exercise, called the Purifying Breath. Do not repeat it more than four times during the same session.[5]

If the breathe-and-hold count of four, sixteen, eight feels uncomfortable or forced, try two, eight, four to keep your breathing pattern as normal as possible. Do not try to take in abnormal amounts of air or hold your breath for unusually long periods. Keep your breathing as comfortable as possible within the exercise. Focus on counting with the breaths, and if your mind strays to other things, bring it back to the counting. After completing the sequence four times, return to normal, slow breaths. Be inwardly as still as possible, paying attention to the thoughts that pass through your mind. Notice them and let them go. When you complete this, you will find yourself quiet inside and ready to pick up your pendulum. If the feeling is new to you, notice it and savor it. Once you know what feeling still inside is like, it is easier to continue achieving it.

A different type of meditation, of Tibetan Buddhist origin and highly popular in Wiccan training, is the Tree of Life meditation. This was my first attempt at meditating, and one day after several weeks of trying it, I had my first Kundalini experience—of Light rising from my root to crown, up and out and down in a whoosh of intense sensations and indescribable colors. It looked and felt like the best Fourth of July fireworks I had ever seen. I was outdoors at the time, lying on my back on the grass under an enormous maple tree. Though it didn't happen again for me for a long time, I was sold on the whole idea of meditation. This type of meditation is called a "guided visualization" or "guided journey." Once you are comfortable with doing meditation indoors at your altar, you can try it outdoors in nature, if you can find a place that is safe and comfortable and where you won't be distracted.

Do your usual preparation for meditating, in a quiet room with a closed door and the phone and other electronics turned off. Light your candle. Get comfortable, and do the rocking side to side and forward and back to center yourself. Take a few deep breaths, put your worries away or burn them in the candle flame, and make yourself as quiet inside as you can. If you can keep from falling asleep, you might try this meditation lying down; otherwise, sit in a straight chair with your feet solidly on the floor. Since this is a visualization, try to add all the sensory perceptions to your experience of it, not only the sound of your mind speaking the images. Use visuals, sounds, fragrances, feelings, and lots of colors.

First imagine the most beautiful and magnificent ancient tree that you can picture. It can be a tree that you know or one that you create by your thoughts. Your job in this meditation is to become that ancient tree; take a moment to do so now. A tree's foundation is its network of many deep-growing roots. Imagine your roots going deeper and deeper into the Earth until they connect and join fully with the core of Light at the center of the planet. What color is the core? These roots are your grounding cord; ask that your grounding cord remain connected to the core of the Earth Mother permanently.

Now that you have anchored your roots, draw Light from the core, drinking deeply through all of your roots. What color is the Light, and are the colors changing? Draw it up through your roots and into your tree trunk. Draw the Light through all the branches that sweep upward from your trunk. Keep drawing in the Light until your branches, every one of them, are filled with it. Your large branches become smaller branches, and the smaller branches end in twigs. Make sure the Light fills all of these. At the end of your twigs are green and yellow-green leaves, tiny white (or yellow, red, or pink) flowers, and golden (or purple, orange, or red) fruit. What kind of fruit is on your tree? Draw the Light, moving from your roots, up through all of these. Bathe everything in Light. Fill everything with Light.

When you are filled with Light from the deepest of your roots to the highest of your fruit and flowers, so filled that you can fill no more, see the Light flow from your tree back down to the ground. Watch your fruit, flowers, leaves, and twigs drip and flow in a rainfall of the brightest Light. If the color of the Light changes again, watch it happen. It may change again and again. The Light spills from your treetop and back to the Earth, back to the core of Mother Earth. Your roots draw the Light in and upward again, and the flow of Light rises and returns. Continue the flow for as long as you wish. Then, as you return to your roots at the core of the Earth, stop drawing the Light, and you're done.

Remain quiet for a while before sitting up again or moving. This meditation will leave you feeling clear, calm, energized, and very quiet inside. It's my personal favorite and the favorite of many Witches. Repeat it as often as you choose to use it, as it will teach you the skill of psychic visualization. It will also cleanse, clear, balance, and open your Kundalini chakras and entire Kundalini energy system. It will help to prepare you for all forms of psychic work, including using a pendulum.

The goal of meditation is to induce an altered state, a state of enhanced awareness. Our thought processes operate in different ways on different levels. For example, what we perceive in sleep is far different from what we perceive in the waking state. When our everyday beta brain waves shift to the slower alpha level, our creativity and concentration are engaged. We can go yet deeper into the theta state, a very slow state used in hypnosis. Sleep is the delta state and slower still. Meditation induces and controls these states, taking us from the everyday beta into the creative alpha and sometimes deeper. These levels of awareness and the means of reaching them are well known and well understood in the East, while Westerners flounder with drugs to induce what they can't create in their own minds. Meditation is better than any drug. It gives you well-being, self-awareness, inner peace, and communication with the Light. And it's legal, nonfattening, and nonaddictive.

Your concentration on the candle flame or bowl of water—or on the counting or the tree—develops the focused mind, though you may not be aware of it while you are intent on emptying your thoughts. Using a pendulum effectively does not require the totally quiet mind of traditional Eastern meditation, but it does require the ability to focus on one point, and all of the above forms of meditation develop both. If you wish to develop your psychic abilities this is the route to travel.

If it is difficult for Westerners to make their minds fully still, and to keep them still for any length of time, developing the focused mind is easier. The focused mind is what is needed for pendulum use. In this case, instead of emptying your mind completely, you empty it of everything except what you are concentrating on. In the meditations above, the concentration can be on the flame or bowl of water, your breathing, or the tree. In working with a pendulum, you concentrate on the tool itself, which will make your mind still enough and clear enough for the reception and transmission of information that you seek.

Go into your quiet room again, close the door, unplug the phone, and light a candle. Bring a pendulum with you into the room and place it in front of you. Don't lie down this time, but sit comfortably; if you are on a chair, your feet should be flat on the floor. Don't cross your arms or your legs. Do the preliminary grounding and centering exercises. Look steadily at the candle flame or bowl of water and focus upon it. Rock your body slowly forward and back, and then from side to side a couple of times without twisting, and then come back to the middle and sit straight and still. Put each of your worries into the candle flame or water or imaginary box, and let them go. Make your breathing slow, deep, and steady. Sit still for a moment, looking at the flame, and calm your mind as much as you can in a few breaths.

Pick up your pendulum by the bead at the top, with the pendant hanging free. As always, this should be a cleansed and purified pendulum, one you have dedicated to the Light. Invite the Light to be with you, and if you know the name of the Light-being who runs your pendulum, invite her to come in. Never command a Be-ing of the Light; you may only invite her (but what is not of the Light, you may command to leave). Remember to say "please" and "thank you," and to be truly grateful for what you receive. Your first two pendulum questions are to ask if the pendulum is absolutely energetically cleared and to ask if your Light-being (or any Be-ing of the Highest Light) is there.

The trick here is to keep your mind completely free of all thoughts other than the question you are asking. Focus your eyes steadily upon your pendulum and hold it in a relaxed way. If thoughts other than your question come, notice them, let them go, and return to what you are asking. You will notice that when your mind drifts away from focusing on your question, your pendulum will react. It might swing "no," or go into a small, slow circle. It could give you any form of response that you know is not the answer to your inquiry. Use the pendulum to ask other questions, one at a time, keeping your mind carefully focused on each one as you ask it. Keep your mind focused on the question until you receive and understand the response. Only then go to your next question.

You can ask for information that you need for yourself, or, as I like very much to do, you can ask your Light-being metaphysical questions or questions about Herself. She will usually be very glad to answer. Remember that with a pendulum you can only receive "yes" or "no" responses; you will learn with experience how to phrase your questions to give you the most information (chapter seven discusses this further). Spend a few minutes each day (ten minutes in the morning and ten at bedtime are good for this too) working with your pendulum. As you practice keeping the one-pointed focus, it gets easier, and the daily pendulum use is also good practice. Eventually you will be able to achieve the one-pointed focus without the candle, meditation, or meditation-type preparation. When you are doing very serious pendulum work, however, and you need the best possible means of communication, doing it in this more structured way is always highly positive.

If you continue these exercises, you will learn to shift your awareness simply and quickly from your daily state to the quiet (or quieter) mind and concentrated focus. This takes a while to happen, but if you do the work, it will. Once it happens, you can shift to the meditative one-pointed focus any time you want. It will eventually happen automatically, as soon as you pick up a pendulum. At this stage, you have learned to change the radio station from that of earth-plane living to the channel for communication with the Light. Your work with the pendulum will become highly meaningful.

Once the meditative state becomes automatic, you may find that you are going deeper into an altered state than you realize. Be very careful to do this only in a safe place. Don't do it while driving, for example, or in any other situation that requires your full attention. (Again, do as I say and not as I do; most of my friends won't ride in the car if I'm driving!) Do this tuning-in automatically every time you start to use a pendulum. Don't cross your arms or legs, as doing so blocks the free flow of energy. If you are not sure about whether the request you are about to make is information you are permitted to have, you can ask before you make the request.

Don't use the pendulum where your lack of attention will get you into trouble, such as at work or school. I have a small friend who is a very spiritual child. When he was about six or seven years old, I made him a pendulum and he learned easily how to use it. It had a blue plastic bead on the top and a teddy bear charm for the swinging weight. (His brother's pendulum had a large sheriff's star for the pendant.) Josh used his pendulum for everything and anything, including asking for right answers in his homework. After that worked, he took it to school. Just as he was asking the pendulum if he would get into trouble for using it in school, his teacher confiscated it. There is a right and wrong place for everything.

One other thing that the one-pointed focused mind requires is that you have no expectations. If you can achieve this, it will keep your own mind from interfering with the accuracy of your responses. Since transmission of information through your pendulum happens by way of your mind, if you have your mind already made up before you ask the question, you will get the answer you expect. If you can keep your mind still and empty, or at least neutral, and focus on the pendulum and your question (instead of on the answer you haven't yet received), your information will be less tainted and much more accurate. It's hard to talk when someone else is talking, and it's hard for your Light-being to tell you something if you are already telling it to yourself—right or wrong.

Give your Light-being the chance to give you the real answer by keeping your mind still and open to the information. Along with your mind, you must also keep your emotions neutral, or again you will taint the results. Some people believe that a pendulum says anything you want it to. If you allow your emotions to interfere, and your mind is not still and focused, that's exactly what will happen. Our desires and emotions are very strong. The meditation exercises that teach you to hold your mind empty and open will also teach you to keep your emotions and opinions from interfering with the information the Light is trying to give you.

Another suggestion—in fact it's a requirement in using the meditative state to enhance your ability to work with a pendulum and the Light—is to work for the good of all. In your meditation sessions with the pendulum, you can ask for healing for the planet or for help for anyone who needs it, including yourself, of course. One outgrowth of a consistent meditation practice is that you develop compassion and love for all of life. This is a good attitude to have, particularly for someone who wishes to work with Light-beings. In everything you do, with a pendulum or anything else, do it with love for yourself, the Light, and all things.

How to Use a Pendulum

It is highly unusual for the detailed "how to do it" chapter to come so late in a book on pendulums or anything else. There is a reason for the delay, however, since the preliminary preparations are so important and may actually be of more importance than the pendulums themselves. By employing these preparations, you make your pendulum into a psychic tool of greater worth and accuracy than most people have ever seen. I use pendulums differently from anyone else I know, and I know that these preliminary foundations are necessary. I use pendulums for healing, including planetary and beyond-planetary healing, for psychic work and psychic readings of all kinds, and to obtain every kind of ethical information. I use them for important things and for less important things—for shopping large and small, for example—and for every kind of choice. The pendulum has become my most important psychic tool. I can depend on its accuracy in virtually every situation and use.

I have dedicated myself and all of my pendulums to the Light, along with everything else that I use, live with, or do. I make very sure that when I use a pendulum it is absolutely energetically cleared and that a Be-ing of the Highest Light and *only* the Highest Light is working through it. I have learned to focus in a concentrated and open-minded way, to keep my opinions and emotions from interfering, and have learned to quiet my mind at least some of the time. My accuracy with the pendulum is about 95 percent, possibly more, which I'm told is far greater than most people who use them can achieve or expect. After all, it's only a button on a string.

The skills taught in the preceding chapters of this book will give you high accuracy with your pendulums, as well as protect you from interference by entities not of the Light. Low-level Be-ings like to play with psychic tools—pendulums, Ouija boards, and even tarot cards—if you allow them to. They don't have your good at heart, only the malicious game of seeing how far they can mislead or confuse you. Some can actually be evil, and I have met and had to deal with entirely too many that are. Pendulums are easy to take over in this way, and dedication and cleansing usually prevent it. The methods in this book establish your pendulum as a tool of the Light, one that works only for the Light, which the Light can use and work through safely.

We have discussed the power of the creative mind and why having a quiet, neutral, one-pointed focus is important. For the first exercise on how to use a pendulum, I'd like to show you more about that. Even though I am just beginning to give directions on how to use pendulums, you may well have come to this book already familiar with them and are already using them. If you have never used pendulums until now, you have probably read ahead to this chapter. If you have done the work of the previous chapters you are now ready to use your pendulum as a tool of the Light. Even if you are already experienced with the pendulum, a lot of this book and its methods and exercises will still be new to you. It will benefit you to add them to the methods you already use, and there may be some current methods that you will wish to change.

For this first exercise session, and at any other time you wish to, use the formal meditation preparations. Go into a quiet room alone, center yourself and let go of your worries, light a candle, and clear your mind. Make sure your pendulums are cleared before you start, and place them ready in front of you. Only use those pendulums that are dedicated to the Light. Invite the Light-being who runs your pendulum for and with you to join you. Do a few minutes of meditation, of whatever kind you prefer, to clear your mind and to focus your intent. You will only work for a few minutes this first time, probably no more than twenty minutes or half an hour, if you even work that long.

Pick up your pendulum and hold it suspended in front of you. Hold it in your right hand if you are right-handed, and in your left hand if you are left-handed. Use a light grip and keep your hand and all of your body relaxed; your preliminary meditation should leave you in a relaxed and calm state. Hold your pendulum between your thumb and first finger by the bead at the top, letting the weight drop straight down. If your pendulum chain is too long, you may feel more comfortable holding it further down the chain, and it is fine to do that. If the pendulum is swinging, stop it with your hand for now and let it hang straight and still.

Clear your mind of all thoughts and focus your eyes on the pendulum weight. Ask if your Be-ing of the Highest Light is with you. Wait for your response. Next ask if she or he is willing to do pendulum work with you at this time. Wait again. Then ask if the pendulum you are holding is absolutely energetically cleared. All three answers should be "yes" before you proceed any further. If your Light-being is not willing to work with you now, ask if there is something she wants you to do first. What that may be will come into your mind. Do what is needed and come back. If she wishes for you to start this work at a different time, do so; you will probably know when and why. Only do this work when your Light-being is ready (which means when she or he feels that you are ready) and if your pendulums are dedicated and cleared.

If you have never used a pendulum before, you'll need to first establish your "yes," "no," and "maybe" responses, and then move on to your questions. The pendulum hanging straight down and without motion is in the "search mode." This means that the pendulum and your mind are in a neutral, waiting state, ready for your question or directions. If your mind is still, the pendulum will hang still. If your mind is not still, quiet it by focusing on the pendulum without allowing chatter or questions to fog your mind. If you need to do the meditation process of noticing your thoughts and releasing them, do so. When you need to do this, it is because you are not fully relaxed, and it is your anxiety that prevents you from being ready. Waiting means to be in readiness and that's what the "search mode" is.

Now, while looking at and focusing on your pendulum, form clearly in your mind the word "yes." Think "yes." Say "yes" silently in your mind, say it again and again and again, slowly and repeatedly. Watch what your pendulum does without stopping its motion. What your pendulum is doing is showing you what a "yes" response will be in all of your pendulum work from here forward. Keep thinking "yes"; it's fun to watch the pendulum move. You will realize that you aren't doing it, but that your mind is doing it, that the pendulum is doing it itself. Actually your Be-ing of the Highest Light has a hand in it, and she is learning to work with you while you are learning how to use the tool.

If nothing happens here, it's because you either haven't made contact with a Light-being, you aren't looking at the pendulum, or you aren't saying "yes" in your mind. Don't say it out loud; say it silently inside your head, focusing your mind on your pendulum and its movement as you do so. This may not work if you aren't relaxed, because if you are too anxious, you are allowing your own mind to interfere. If you want it to happen too much, you stimulate the anxiety. Just remember that anyone can do this, and you will too, so don't stress it. Try *imagining* you can do it, and you will suddenly be doing it. You can do anything you can imagine, and to imagine is to visualize—a powerful psychic skill of its own. I've taught lots of small children to use pendulums—they love the kinds that are made from hardware bolts and washers on colored string. If they can learn this, so can you.

The strength of the pendulum's swing may be very small and weak at the beginning, but it will get stronger and more decisive with practice. You and your Be-ing of the Light have to learn to work together; she has to learn how to influence your subconscious to move your neuromuscular system and the pendulum itself. If this is a Light-being who has never run a pendulum before, it will take her some time to get used to it, as it will take you some time to gain expertise in a new psychic ability. If the pendulum moves at all, that's enough for now. Notice what the swing is doing and what it looks like when you say "yes." This response is, and always will be, your "yes" response.

Now do the same thing again, but this time think "no." Think it repeatedly, with all other thoughts cleared from your mind. Don't forget to relax, and don't forget to look at the pendulum while doing this. Occasionally someone's "no" response is simply that—no response. If your pendulum stays still and doesn't move at all, that may be your indication of the answer "no." Keep thinking "no" until you have established what your "no" will look like. Try "yes" and "no" again a few times. You may be getting tired by this time (it's amazing how using your brain can make you tired!), but we are nearly done with this first session.

The next thing you need to do is to establish how your pendulum responds when the answer is neutral or uncertain. This is the non-answer of "maybe." It can mean "I don't know," or "Give me more information," or "There is no answer at this time," or "This is not information you may have." In my own pendulum work, I get a neutral response plus one other, different response. If I'm on the right track and whoever is working with me wants me to keep thinking or analyzing on the subject, my pendulum does a wildly gyrating circular swing. You may or may not develop such a response, but you probably won't have it at the beginning. Establish your neutral swing by looking at the pendulum, clearing your mind, and focusing on it as you did for the "yes" and "no." This time the word to think and say in your mind repeatedly is "maybe." Observe what this swing looks like, and try the "yes" and "no" again as well.

Now, invite your Be-ing of the Highest Light to join with you on the last part of this exercise. So far you have used your own mind, but now you will join your thoughts with that of your Light-being. Hold your pendulum still in the "search mode," clear your mind of all thoughts, and look at your pendulum. Ask of your Be-ing of the Highest Light, "Please show me 'yes.'" Clear your mind completely and wait and watch your pendulum's response. This time your pendulum will move, in the same swing as indicated "yes" before, but now you will be very aware that someone other than you is moving it. You are doing nothing but holding still in a relaxed way and letting your Light-being do the work. Remember to say "thank you."

Once the "yes" is established, ask your Be-ing of the Highest Light, "Please show me a 'no.'" Again clear your mind completely, focus your eyes on the pendulum, and observe the response. You will feel your hand being moved, and the pendulum will swing. Do the same thing again for the "maybe." Ask to see the "yes," "no," and "maybe" again, repeating a few times until you really get the feel of it, and then stop. Thank your Be-ing of the Light and end the session. This is enough for the first time, but try it again the next day. You may feel more tired than you would expect, and you may feel spacey. Put down the pendulum and place your hands on the floor for a few minutes to ground yourself and clear the energy. Put your pendulum into salt or under your pyramid to clear. If you feel hungry, look for something with protein in it to eat; a few bites are enough. Avoid sugar, though that may be what you think you crave. I like to eat a piece of cheese or spoonful of cottage cheese at this time.

Here is a fun exercise for making a pendulum move with your mind. One of the apartments I used to live in was on two floors, the second and third floors above a pizza shop. Inside the apartment, there was a curved flight of carpeted stairs between the two floors. The stairs had an open-rung wooden railing on one side and the wall on the other. I could hang something on a long string from a rung at the top of the stairwell, and the object would dangle in the center of a step near the bottom of the flight. At the bottom of the string, I tied a faceted lead-crystal feng shui ball, a little more than an inch in diameter and about an inch and a half high. When I walked downstairs, there was a step upon which I was facing the ball at just above eye level. Sometimes coming down, I would stand on the step and coax the ball to move with my mind. It was a game I got fairly good at. I could make it swing back and forth or even side to side.

(You can do this with a candle flame too. Determine "yes" and "no" with the moving flame and use it as a pendulum!) It's a game that might help you learn to focus your mind for pendulum work.

The next day, or the next time that you wish to work, repeat the first session's exercises again. It will be much quicker and easier the second time, and it will get even easier with more days of practice. Once you have joined with your Be-ing of the Light and reviewed again your "yes," "no," and "maybe" pendulum swings, begin asking some questions of your pendulum and Light-being. Start with questions to which you already know the answers. Try them first using your own mind, with the answer spoken in your mind running the pendulum's response, and then try them with your mind held clear and your Light-being giving the response. Such simple and obvious questions might be something like, "Is my name Jane?" "Do I live with a dog?" "Is it Tuesday?" These are all questions with obvious answers, but they are all you need for a start.

Once you are confident that the obvious questions are receiving correct answers, you can try some less obvious ones. Begin to ask for real information. Note, however, that whatever your questions are now or will be later, whether they are obvious or not, it doesn't serve to ask facetious questions, sarcastic ones, or questions that have no reasonable answers. Don't try to trick your Light-being with your questions, and don't ask her for information that you have no reason to want to know. Your Light-being won't understand—Light-beings are almost always very innocent—and your lack of respect will not help your relationship with her.

If a Be-ing of the Light thinks you are being disrespectful, she will withdraw. If you are always disrespectful, she may decide not to work with you. Don't hurt her feelings, which you might too easily do. Remember, you also may not give her commands; only ask or invite her, and she will readily cooperate. Treat her always with the greatest consideration and respect, and your relationship will be more loving and rewarding than anything you can imagine. Have gratitude and express it.

Remember that you have an equal part in this partnership with a Being of the Highest Light. You are a Light-being in training yourself. Our spiritual job and purpose for being on Earth is to evolve ourselves into the Light-beings we were meant to be. This means learning love and compassion, along with the knowledge and understanding of who we are and how things spiritually work. If you have been granted Highest Light guidance, it means that you are well on your way. You are on the path to Ascension/Enlightenment, and that a Light-being is helping you means that you have the potential to succeed. Your responsibility is what it always has been—to be the very best that you can be and to do your best to serve goodness and the Light in every way that you can. Your evolution is for yourself, but in the law of critical mass, it is also for everyone else.

None of this means that you can't have fun along the way, and it is truly important to do so. I always feel in anything I do or teach that if it's not fun, I'm not doing my job. What is serious can usually be fun, and it very often needs to be. I do lots of pendulum work that is quite serious and even sometimes dangerous. But Brede also likes to run my pendulum to pick things out of shopping catalogs to buy. I tease Her that She's the Goddess of shopping and chocolate, and give Her everything I can that She asks for. There is a bumper sticker that says, "Angels fly because they take themselves lightly," and it's true. You can do your work and do it in a serious and responsible way, but with most things, you can also have fun while doing it.

When working with any of your pendulums and with all Be-ings of the Highest Light, the "yes," "no," and non-answer of "maybe" code that you have established will never change. No matter who may run your pendulums with you now or in the future, and no matter which of many pendulums you may borrow, buy, or make, the responses stay the same. It's your permanent binary code, and few people will have one exactly like yours. For me, "yes" is a vertical up-and-down motion and "no" is a counterclockwise circle. A "maybe" is a very small version of "no." Your pendulum's responses will probably not be the same as mine, and they probably won't be like those of anyone else you know. Your responses will be established for the workings of your own mind and neurological system. Everyone is different. There is no right or wrong here, only what works. As long as you can interpret what the responses mean, it's all that you need.

Your pendulum can swing in a straight line, circle in either direction, and give you small or large swings. It can spin (sometimes wildly), and it can hold still. Don't try to change the code you've been assigned, there is no reason ever to do so. If your pendulum's swing seems so small that you can't interpret it, try lengthening the chain or cord by an inch or two, which will automatically give you a wider swing. Or ask your Light-being to increase the size of the swing so that you can more easily interpret it. If you are having any other difficulty, ask your Be-ing of the Light for help, and together you will resolve any problems. Remember that you are working in a partnership and not alone.

Once you are comfortable with the parameters of the responses, and you are comfortable working in partnership with your Light-being, start asking more complex questions. You might start with questions that have answers you don't know but can easily find out. Ask your questions and then check on the answers, verifying the accuracy of what you've been given. Once you are comfortable with these types of questions, you can start asking questions for real information, inquiring about things that you don't know but want to know about or need to know. You will learn to trust the accuracy of the responses and to trust your partnership with the Light-being who has chosen to work with you. By the time you have done all this and become experienced, you will have a real idea of what a pendulum can do and how to use it.

There are times when you should not use a pendulum for information because you will not be able to trust the responses. The problems always originate with you. These times are usually when your emotions or preconceived thoughts interfere with your Light-being's ability to communicate clearly with you and to give you valid information. If you are highly

DIAGRAM 1

PENDULUM SWINGS

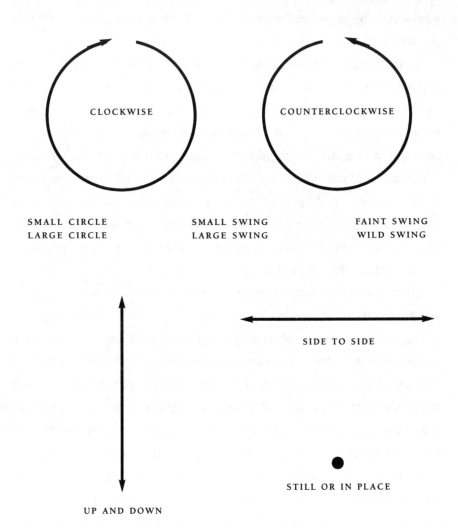

CLOCKWISE

COUNTERCLOCKWISE

SMALL CIRCLE
LARGE CIRCLE

SMALL SWING
LARGE SWING

FAINT SWING
WILD SWING

SIDE TO SIDE

STILL OR IN PLACE

UP AND DOWN

These are the ways that a pendulum can swing. Use your
mind to cause the pendulum to swing in these figures.
One at a time, hold the pendulum over the center of each
diagram and ask it to "Follow the line on the diagram."

emotional about something and therefore unable to keep your mind neutral, it's best not to use the pendulum. Wait until you calm down and are more in control before you ask about the situation. Never force the answers to your questions or try to make them into what you think they ought to be.

Some situations may be so charged for you that you can never ask, as you will never get a clear response, and in those cases it's best to find someone else to do the asking. Get a tarot or psychic reading done by a reliable practitioner who is not emotionally involved. If you are angry, don't use the pendulum; you will not be able to trust the information, and your anger may draw to you entities that are not of the Light. Your own Be-ing of the Highest Light will withdraw from your anger as well. Don't use the pendulum if you are too distracted to focus properly, or too upset or ill to focus and to keep a neutral mind.

Never use the pendulum or do psychic work of any kind when you are under the influence of alcohol or recreational drugs. These substances impair your judgment and can affect your sense of appropriateness and responsibility. This is the time when you are most likely to push for answers you are not ethically supposed to have. If your mind is not functioning at its best, your neurological system won't be either. The pendulum either won't work or will give you false responses. Your Light-being also may refuse to work through your pendulums when you are under the influence of a negative substance. Such substances can put you and your Be-ing of the Highest Light in danger from low- level entities, discarnate spirits (ghosts), negative elementals, attachments, and more.

An entity drawn to you in this way could harm you and your Light-being. If you or your pendulums are taken over by such energies, your Light-being cannot return until both you and your pendulum are cleansed, purified, and healed of any damage. Such entities do negative and evil things that are not easy to heal and that cause much suffering. You have a responsibility to protect your Be-ing of the Highest Light. Why take the risk for her or for yourself?

There are some questions that you will want to make frequent use of in your pendulum work. These will help you know whether you are requesting information that you should (or shouldn't) be asking for. Use your pendulum to ask, and always allow your Light-being to guide you. Obey the "no." You are already familiar with two of these questions. They are "Is this pendulum absolutely energetically cleared?" and "Is a Be-ing of the Highest Light [use her name once you know it] running this pendulum?" Here are a few more that will be of help. "May I?" or "Am I permitted?" is a big one. If the request is something you are not sure you have the right to make, you can find out by asking this. If the answer is "no," drop the subject. "Should I?" is another good question. You might be permitted, but is it the best thing to do? Some things are better not to know. If you suspect that someone you care about is dying, do you want to know? Do you want to know when?

"Can I?" is another such reality check. You might want to do something or ask for something and it might be permitted. But is it possible? Is it something you can accomplish? Some limits just can't be pushed—and, believe me, I've tried to push them all! There are some things you just can't do, though there aren't very many of them. But if you can't, perhaps there is a Be-ing of the Highest Light who *can* do them. If the request is worthy, you might ask if there is someone who can (and is willing) to do what you need, and if it is permitted to ask them to do it. Another such question might be, "Would it be for the best good to ask this?" Sometimes it is and sometimes it isn't. Follow the guidance of your Light-being and trust her.

One other such question can be a useful reality check when you're not sure that something is true. Ask your Light-being by way of your pendulum, "Is this the truth?" or "Is this really so?" Very often you can discern truth from fiction, a lie from what's real, by asking this question. Sometimes what you think is real or true might not be, and asking can save you from a bad situation or from doing something you'd be sorry for later. Another inquiry along these lines is, "Is it for the highest good?" or

"Is it for the good of all?" This should be the final deciding criterion for every request you make and everything you do. It is the ultimate truth, and if your request passes this test, you're home free.

In every request when using the pendulum, your goal should be to determine what is absolutely true. Truth is not always what you wish it to be, but truth is what is. Finding truth is your job and what a pendulum is for. It's not a place where wishful thinking can be allowed to enter. This is why you work so hard to keep your mind clear, your emotions neutral, and your thoughts from interfering. Anyone can make things up as they go along. Anyone can make the pendulum say anything they want it to say. But what's the point? What have you gained and how have you grown by doing that? If you don't want the truth or can't handle the truth, don't ask the question.

Wiccans use an ethic that seems simplistic but that is really quite exacting. It is just this: "Harm none." Life is filled with every possibility. Earth is a smorgasbord of delights and choices. If what you do harms none, including yourself and the planet, you are free to do anything you want, to sample any dish on the table. But if something is at risk of harming anything—human or nonhuman—it is not to be thought of, much less done. And this has to include yourself. Harming none begins with you.

The Wiccan religion has another ethic, or "rede" as they are called, another rule to live by. This one is simple also, with as wide an application as the one above. This one says, "What you send out comes back to you." Some Witches say it comes back to you threefold. Other Witches say it returns tenfold. Either way, this ethic is a reminder to be very careful about what you do, for the results will rebound upon you. If you do good, good comes back to you multiplied. If you do wrong, likewise. The rule covers both actions and thoughts. What we think, we create, and "Thoughts are things" is another adage. All Creation begins with thought, and Creation is thought made manifest. You may say to this that you are just a person in body and that Creation is for the Goddesses and Gods. This is so in the big things, but in the smaller ones of our own lives, we are often able to create some part of our lives ourselves. This is not to say that if something goes wrong, it's all your fault and you caused it—that's not always so. But what it is saying is that you have power in your thoughts and actions that can maximize your potential. Use those thoughts wisely to maximize the good things, the things that you want for yourself and you want in your service to the Light. Understand that you and your thoughts have consequences, and create accordingly. Let everything you do and think be something that you would not be ashamed or afraid to have returned to you.

Remember these adages and redes in all of your dealings with the Being of the Highest Light that has chosen to run the pendulum with you. That relationship, if nurtured and treated responsibly, can grow. The Earth is on an Ascension path, and so are many of those who live here. Many women and a few men will be chosen to bring in a Goddess or a God to join with them fully, as Brede has done with me. Some people, in addition, will bring in a Family of Light, a group of Light-beings to work through them. Let your work with the pendulum be the beginning of a path of Ascension and Light that could bring a Goddess or a God to live with you. It is not impossible; it has happened for many people already, and there will be many more. The Light does the choosing, and the Be-ings of the Light who come here decide whom they want to be joined with. There is no reason that it can't be you, if you are willing to be all you can be and to serve the Light.

Your pendulum is a tool that will help you to maximize your service to the Light, and that service will come back to you tenfold. Use it wisely and well and with joy, but also with responsibility and great love.

How to Ask Questions

Pendulums can only convey "yes" or "no" responses, along with the non-answer of "maybe." Your questions have to be phrased in such a way that "yes" or "no" gives you all the information you need and is the whole answer. This is not the way we normally ask questions and gain information, or receive meaningful answers, so asking in this way is a new skill to learn. The degree to which your pendulum is useful depends in large part on how well you learn this skill and how consistently you apply it. Once you have learned the language, however, the information you can obtain using a pendulum run by a Be-ing of the Highest Light is virtually limitless.

The high technology of our modern culture is primarily based upon the computer. Computers pervade our lives for every possible use, from medical to entertainment. They are sources of information on every possible subject; they are whole libraries in a box. Today's children learn computers before they even learn to read, and their expertise extends beyond that of most adults. They are growing up with computers and computer languages, and they understand them and know how to use them. While these children may reject the tools and skills that have been important to older generations, they are establishing a culture of their own, based upon technologies not available even just a few years ago.

There is an analogy here with pendulums, which are the very simplest of computers. Computers, for all the vast information they obtain and store, operate on the binary code system. This is a two-based, one or two, on or off, yes or no coding, which is similar to Braille or to the older Morse telegraph code's dots and dashes, and is used to create a limitless language. Every piece of information in a computer, every computer function, is comprised of binary codes, of "yes" or "no." And it is only of "yes" or "no." Computers are very close in function to human brains. The clearest analogy of how Creation operates is as a computer, or as a series of computers, which are also the Creational Minds of the Light. If the "yes" or "no" system works for the computers that run our technology and also works for Creation, we can make it work for us with the pendulum.

As people who run the computers, however, we are not used to speaking or thinking in a technology with only two possibilities. Computer binary functions are retranslated into our language. Pendulums can only give us two possibilities, and we have to learn a new form of language to use them. Such language may seem awkward at first, but once learned, you have the key to a great deal of information. Like learning to use a computer, learning the language of pendulums opens a lot of informational doors. Also as with the computer, our input errors bring about errors in the output. By learning to work with the pendulum binary language, you reduce and prevent many errors and greatly increase the quality of what you receive.

One of the most frequent reasons why pendulums don't seem to work, or don't work accurately and usefully, is because the questions asked of them are not phrased (thought) in a language that can yield an accurate response. Your questions have to have a "yes" or "no" answer; there is no way to get around this. They have to be phrased very simply and without ambiguity of any kind. A clear question gets a clear answer; an unclear question gets an unclear or wrong answer. "Garbage in, garbage out," as they say with computers. Your job is to ask cleanly and clearly, and without any garbage in your thoughts at all.

We are back to thought here, as it is the raw material of every aspect of Creation—and of computers, psychic abilities, and pendulum use. Thought is the sole means of transmitting information between your mind and that of your Light-being's. The pendulum is the reception tool, the means of registering the Light-being's response. It is only a tool and it can only register what it receives—exactly what it receives. The pendulum itself does not think. What the tool receives is a response to your question, which is made, sent, received, and registered by way of thought. The response that is given to you is based totally upon what you ask—exactly and precisely what you ask. What you ask for is what you will receive. Your Light-being can't or won't edit your questions to give you what you *intend;* she will only respond to exactly what you ask.

Why? The Light is of far higher sentience than we are and certainly more highly evolved. Light-beings have technology and creative abilities we can't even imagine. Their knowledge, and their ability to obtain knowledge from each other, from us, and from the Collective Consciousness, is limitless. Be-ings of the Light have a Collective Consciousness of their own; what one knows everyone knows. All information is shared and known to all, and if someone needs to know something, she has the resources to find out about anything she wishes. Their intelligent minds are far beyond anything we can do with computers or with our own limited minds and brains. So, are our Light-beings willfully frustrating us? No.

Light-beings are only ethically permitted to answer what we ask, and answer exactly what we ask. This is because we must achieve our evolution step-by-step, taking each step only when we are ready for it. If we ask a question, especially about how the Cosmos works, it is because we are evolved to the point where we are ready to know. If we are not ready to know, it is considered unethical to tell us. It would only confuse us, like teaching geometry to a child in kindergarten. Every Be-ing of the Light who runs our pendulums or provides teaching in any other way is bound to obey this evolutionary law. This law extends to our guidance on all levels and in such things as channeling, psychic readings, healing, tarot, and all other psychic work.

The law allows the sometimes tantalizing information that the Light puts into our minds to stimulate our questions. The questions are planted because we are ready for them. They lead us forward when it is time to do so. Evolutionary laws have karmic consequences, and to violate them would be for a Light-being to violate our karma. Potential harm could result to us. The rule of evolutionary law was made by our Creator Nada, and no Be-ing of the Light will disobey it. Nor should we ask Light-beings to or want them to—it's for our own good. Sometimes a little information in the wrong place or time can be a dangerous thing.

Having to know what to ask is also a discipline, an evolutionary discipline. As each question takes us forward step-by-step on our learning path, the discipline teaches us to analyze and think. Like a computer tutorial that only lets the student go forward when she has mastered the current lesson, our having to ask for what we want to know is part of the means by which we learn. This learning is a major aspect of our spiritual growth. It is a part of the evolution of our Be-ing, and with critical mass, our evolution becomes that of all Be-ings. It has to be done right, which means that we have to learn each lesson entirely before moving to the next lesson. Our questions reflect what we have already learned. They are the bridge between what we know now and what we are ready to know next.

The thoughtfulness (break down the word to its meaning—thought-full-ness) of your questions directly reflects where you are on your evolutionary path. If you are asking questions that are thoughtless (again break down the word to its meaning—thought-less) you are not yet ready to go forward. *Why* do you want to know what you are asking? Is it out of wanting to pry into another's life? Or is it for the purpose of evolving yourself to serve others and the Light? There is a world of difference here. Curiosity stimulates knowledge and fosters your growth and evolution. It is to be encouraged—as long as the purposes are ethical. Every question is a step in the development of your mind and thought; evolution is the development of your mind. Remember that what you think, you also create, and that what you create has consequences.

Because of this, to develop and evolve your mind and spirituality, you must ask your Light-being precisely what you wish to know. She can only answer what you ask and can only answer it exactly. And since she has to answer indirectly through your pendulum, a "yes" or "no" answer is all that she can give you. You must learn to phrase your questions so that "yes" or "no" gives you as much information as possible. Remember to stay focused, emotionally neutral, and with your mind clear while you form the question in your mind and with your thoughts. Remember to look at the pendulum until you have your answer. The rest is in how to frame the questions themselves.

To use a pendulum effectively, your questions must be short and simply phrased. It may require a series of several "yes" or "no" questions to give you the answer to one question in all of its parts. You can ask of your Light-being, "Do you love me?" (and the answer will always be "yes"). But you *can't* ask her, "*Why* do you love me?" unless you ask her a series of questions using all the possible reasons why she might love you. "Is it because I'm nice?" "Is it because you love everyone?" "Is it because I'm worthy of your love?" You will probably get a "yes" to all of these, but they may or may not answer the "why?"

Short questions are easiest to phrase and less likely to have the possibility of dual answers. Watch for the words "and" and "or" in your requests. Question like, "Is this a robin or a mockingbird?" won't give you a valid answer. Try it like this: "Is this a robin?" "Yes" or "no." "Is it a mockingbird?" "Yes" or "no." If both are "no," ask, "Is it neither?" If it's neither, you might ask more questions naming other types of birds until you find which one it really is. Where there is an "or" or "and" in your question, you will usually need to break it into two questions. Ask each question one at a time, and wait for the first response before asking for the second. If you are asking one question while thinking ahead to the next, you may get the answer to the second question instead of the first. Keep your mind and thoughts clear, and think only of the question or piece of it that you are asking for right now.

Another example of incorrect phrasing is "Should I buy this necklace or the other one?" The correct phasing is "Should I buy this necklace?"

Look at it or touch it while you are making the inquiry. Receive the response, and then ask, "Or should I buy the other necklace?" Look at that one now, or touch it while you ask. Your next questions on the subject might be, "Is there a necklace different from both of these that I should buy?" Or "Would it be best to buy both?" "Would it be best not to buy any of these necklaces?" Hold your mind steady as you think of each question; if you repeat it in your mind, don't change the wording, as doing so could change your response.

If you know the party game of "Twenty Questions," it's a good exercise for learning to phrase pendulum inquiries. In this game, one person thinks of an object, and the others playing have to guess what the object is. The players can ask up to twenty questions about the object, and the one who guesses it correctly wins. The person thinking of the object has to answer truthfully but can only answer "yes" or "no." If after twenty questions, no one has guessed correctly, the game ends without a winner. Try a few rounds of this. It will help immensely in teaching you how to ask pendulum questions in a way that will give you the most information.

If you ask serious pendulum questions, and ask them in a serious way, you will get a proper response. Ask of your pendulum and Light-being only what you actually want to know. If you don't care, why bother? Your lack of caring will not gain you a legitimate answer. Your Light-being may not understand a joke (though Light-beings are always ready for fun), and she will not honor a request that even jokingly suggests harm or derision to anyone. What you use the pendulum to ask for indicates your true level of spiritual evolution. Take that into consideration in how you make your requests and in what you ask for. If you honestly want to know something, however, and it harms none and violates no one's privacy or free will, you should ask freely. As you gain more experience in how to phrase clear questions, you will learn how to maximize the information you receive.

When you are given an answer to your inquiry, accept it as it's given, whether it's the answer you wanted or not. Don't ask the same question again and again, hoping for a different response. You can ask further questions to clarify the response, but the answer itself is not going to change unless some condition changes or the situation shifts. That will not happen immediately. If you are unsure about the answer, you can ask, "Is this the truth?" If so, it's the truth as it is at this time. You can ask again tomorrow or in a few hours, if you feel the need, but nothing's going to change right away. If you are still in doubt, you might ask, "Do I need to rephrase my question to get a clearer response?" Or, "Is this communication clear?" and "Do I need to make further inquiries about this?" Sometimes you need more information to get a clear response and can ask for it if that's the case. If your question was clear, simple, and unambiguous, however, and you focused properly in asking it, you can and should accept the response. Your Light-being will never lie to you.

Sometimes conditions do change, and your answer can change if that happens. I gave the example of the handyman earlier in this book. My pendulum said that he was coming before three o'clock. When he didn't show up by three o'clock, I asked again, "Is he coming *today?*" and was told no. He had been paged for another job while on his way to my home, and he went there instead. He did come just before three o'clock—the *next* day. This example illustrates two points. First, that your response may be accurate when you ask it but that something can change. Second, that when you are asking about time, you have to make your inquiries very carefully. In my first inquiry, I asked about the time but didn't specify the day.

It is possible to receive accurate information on quantities and amounts with a pendulum. As discussed earlier, time questions are trickier, since time is an Earth-only construct and our Light-beings have difficulty in measuring it. Again, when asking questions regarding time, always specify the day; state that your question is about today or whichever other day you mean. "Will I complete this book today?" "Will I complete it on a Tuesday?" "Will it be next Tuesday?" "Will it be the Tuesday after next?" If you have a calendar, you can first point to today's date and show your Light-being that this is today. Then place your finger on the next Tuesday and ask, "Will I finish the book on this date?"

When you ask the question that gets the "yes," you might ask for *when* on that date. "Will I finish it in the morning?" "Will I finish it by supper time?" "Will I finish it after midnight?" Again, remember that the situation may change. You might be interrupted for some reason or might skip a day's work, and the completion will then take longer than projected. Notice the before-and-after concepts. If you ask, "Will I finish it at two o'clock," and the actual finish time will be two-fifteen, you will get a "no" to your inquiry. If you ask, "Will I finish it before two o'clock?" and you get a "no," next ask, "Will I finish it before three o'clock?" And there's the "yes." If you want the exact time, frame more questions in this way. If it's between two and three o'clock, ask, "Will I finish it before two-thirty?" That's a "yes," so you know it's between two o'clock and two-thirty. If you ask, "Will I finish it before two-fifteen?" and get "no," and then ask, "Will I finish it *at* two-fifteen?" there's the "yes."

My dogs are all rescue animals. When they come to me, I usually don't know their exact ages. I might be given an approximate age by the rescue group or animal shelter, and sometimes those approximate ages are very obviously incorrect. The astrological sign and birth date of a new pet can give me information about the animal that is helpful. When Tiger (the third Tiger) came to me, I was told that she was a year old and that she was very small because she had been badly malnourished. She was terribly thin, but I also suspected that she was much younger than a year old. With pendulum inquiries, I was surprised to find that she was only seven and a half months old. When I questioned the accuracy of this and pulled out a calendar for Brede to show me her birth date, the date She gave me reflected exactly seven and a half months. Full grown now, the dog is still small for a Siberian husky, but she will never again be malnourished. Knowing that she's a Taurus and that Taurus people or animals are stubborn, fastidious homebodies also explains some of her needs to me.

Here is the sequence of requests I made with my pendulum to find Tiger's birth date. First I asked, "Is the dog a year old?" "No." "Is she younger than a year old?" This was "yes." "Is she younger than eleven months old?" "Yes." "Is she younger than ten months old?" "Yes." Counting down, when I asked, "Is she younger than seven months old?" I got a "no" response. Because I questioned the accuracy of this—I didn't think she was that young—I asked Brede, "Is seven and a half months the dog's true age?" The answer was "yes." When I took out the calendar, I started at what would have been nine months, asking, "Is her birth month earlier than this?" "Yes."

When I got a "yes" to the right calendar page and month, I went week by week. "Was the dog born in this week?" "No." When I found the right week by this method, I went day by day until I got a "yes." Then I asked, "Was April 30, 1999, Tiger's correct birth date?" The answer was "yes." Still not convinced that the dog was so young, I asked, "Is this the absolute truth?" When I got a "yes" again, I knew the information was correct.

When making inquiries regarding time, the past is easier to gain accurate information about than the future. What happened in the past has already occurred and is not subject to change. What's coming in the future will very often shift. The future is subject to changing circumstances, to changed minds, and to free will. Though it is possible to ask questions about the future and to do psychic readings that deal with what is to come via the pendulum, it is still an inexact science. When working with the Lords of Karma, they tell me to focus on what is happening in the present and what has already happened in the past, since healing these will change the future automatically by changing the causal conditions. They are reluctant to accept karmic release requests for the future.

Valid prophecy is possible with the pendulum—I do it all the time. It is important, however, to be aware that your accuracy will be lower than usual with questions about the future. This is an aspect of pendulum work to wait for until you are very experienced and until your Be-ing of the Highest Light agrees to undertake it with you. Not all Light-beings will agree to give you future information. If you do this kind of work, be very aware of its limitations. If you do it for others, you are ethically bound to carefully explain to them what its limitations are. When doing this or any psychic work for others, you must also respect confidentiality and privacy. Whatever information you receive for someone other than yourself, you must tell the person what you have learned and tell only the person whom the information is meant for. No one else has the right to know.

In the same ways that you derive time information, you can receive information on amounts, percentages, and quantities—any form of measurement. If you want to know how close something is to completion, you can ask in terms of time or in terms of quantity. Use questions with "more than" or "less than" for these types of measurement questions. Try percentages. "Is the project more than 75 percent complete?" "Yes." "Is it more than 80 percent complete?" "No." So your answer is more than 75 and less than 80 percent. If you want a closer figure, do a series of counting questions until you get the "yes."

Shopping with pendulums is a whole different world. If there is something you want and you ask the pendulum if you should buy it, be very careful to keep your desire and emotion out of your inquiry. If you can keep your mind neutral, you might end up with something even better than what you thought you wanted. Or you might keep yourself from buying something inferior or that doesn't match, or from overspending in a way that you'd later regret. Brede likes to shop, and I give Her free reign on decorating. She picks the towels, wallpaper, furniture, crystals, and everything else I bring home. I have never had cause to regret Her taste, which is usually much better than mine. (Except that She likes red backpacks and suitcases, which She decorates with jingling bells, when my own tastes run to something quieter and blue.)

In a store, I hold a pendulum over the choice of whatever item I'm seeking until I get Brede's approval, a "yes." I can also ask Brede, "Is this too much to spend?" "Can I afford to buy this now?" When Brede first came in fully and I could hear Her through direct communication, She wanted something that I thought was too expensive. I told Her so, and Her response was, "You can give them one of those blue pieces of paper!" I had to explain to Her how a checkbook works and that money has to go in before it comes out. She got the concept, and if She understands it, all of the Light understands it—they have a Collective Consciousness. If your Light-being, through your pendulum, wants you to buy something you'd rather not, the choice has to be yours. (You're the one with the blue pieces of paper, after all.) Use your common sense in this, but have fun with it.

All of the Goddesses, in my experience, like to shop. They think it's wonderful that you can pick something out and bring it home, and they love the variety of what's available in stores. They also love catalogs and think it's even more wonderful to pick something from a book and have it delivered in a few days. Materiality is new to them, and they are curious. As little as we know about their world, they know very little about ours too. Brede constantly finds me bargains, sales, and values. She likes to buy "chocolates in boxes" and to do it after holidays when the candy is half-price. Her reasoning is that if it's half-price we can buy twice as much. Take a pendulum and a Goddess shopping, and you never know what you'll come home with. Some of the Ladies of my Family of Light went shopping with me one day, and we brought home forty-five dollars' worth of candles. None of them thought it was overdoing it!

Your Light-being will draw you to what she's interested in buying. You'll know. Your first pendulum request might be, "Are you interested in looking at this?" Then, "Are you interested in buying one of these?" (She might want more than one.) When Brede has examined all of the possibilities, I go through the shopping cart and ask Her to "show me what we really need to buy now." Then, with the pendulum in my right hand, I touch each object with my left hand, asking, "Do you want to buy this now?" There may be things to put back. I might then ask, "Should we pay by check?" "Should we pay by cash?" She always knows. She has never asked for something that is too expensive or asked when I don't have the money.

Once we went to a big toy store and walked around for hours. Brede had to look at everything, and when I asked what She was looking for, She said that She was "collecting ideas." Finally after the third complete walk-through, She picked a very odd selection of toys. I didn't know what most of them were, but the total cost didn't come to very much, so I humored Her and brought them home. Once they were inside, She told me who was to receive each toy for Solstice (which was more than six months away), except for one item that seemed the strangest of all—a bag of assorted plastic fruit. The fruit was for my dog Kali, who was delighted with toys to tear up. The rest of the items went to friends' children, who all wanted to know how I knew what they really wanted.

One time in the supermarket, Brede wanted a "celebration dinner." She led me first to a container of tabouleh, and I put it in the cart. In the fish department, She wanted something, and I didn't know what it was until She led me with the pendulum to a large, red ready-cooked lobster. I couldn't believe She wanted this, but the pendulum kept swinging a very strong "yes" over it. As I finished my shopping, I asked Her repeatedly, "Can we put this back now?" and the response always was "no." I brought it home, and as I had never eaten lobster, I had to call friends to ask how to do it. While we were eating, I asked Brede, "Why do you want this? You never let me eat anything that looks alive." I haven't eaten meat for twenty years, since Brede's been joined with me, though I do eat fish. This time I could hear Her clearly. "It's okay," She said. "It's just a big bug." She was quite pleased with Her celebration dinner!

When I write books, I have a pendulum in front of me at all times. I use it to ask Brede whether to continue or to stop, to write more on a subject or go on to the next, to move something to another section or page, and whether to add a particular example or not. The pendulum questions might be phrased something like: "Should I stop and take a break now?" "Am I too tired to write more tonight?" "Would this sentence go better with the last paragraph?"

I use the pendulum in editing to ask Brede whether and where to make paragraph breaks, change wording (and what to change it to), add or subtract commas, and sometimes even to help me with spelling. To do this, I focus my mind on what I'm examining and look at the page rather than at the pendulum. I hold the pendulum as I go over each written line. If there's something to be revised, the pendulum swings to "no" as I read it. I look at the word or line and think of how to change it. When the right word or phrase comes into my mind, the pendulum swings to "yes." By the time I have completed a book, Brede has not only channeled it for me, but gone over every line and word to edit it using the pendulum. This is the twenty-fourth book that Brede has written with me this way, and we have learned to work well together.

You will learn to work with your Be-ing of the Highest Light in this co-creative way as well. By trial and error, you will learn how to phrase the questions you use with the pendulum. You will learn what works and what doesn't and what methods are optimal for giving you the information that you need. If you keep in mind that your Be-ing of the Highest Light takes your questions, and every word of your questions, absolutely literally, you'll do fine. You will learn to keep your questions precise and exact, with no ambiguous words or phrases. You will learn to ask one question at a time and keep them simple. As you and your Light-being learn to work together, she will direct you in what questions to ask and how to ask them. The words will seem to come into your mind, whether you actually hear her speaking to you or not.

All it takes is practice, and practice means just that you keep working at it, that you keep using the pendulum. Talk to your Light-being in your mind; she hears you even if her responses come only through the pendulum. Ask for her help and she'll provide it. Treat her with the greatest respect, and treat with respect the information that you gain. Treat the pendulum and your use of it with respect as well. It's a tool that gives you communication with the Light—information, teaching, and so much more.

TROUBLESHOOTING

There is a wide variety of reasons why a pendulum can give you wrong or implausible answers. It is only a tool, and how you use it is crucial. Your Light-being will never be wrong, but she may not be able to give you accurate communication. The purpose of this chapter is to discuss some of the things that go wrong and why, and to look at whatever means of correcting or preventing such problems are possible. As you work with pendulums and your Light-being, you will find occasional times when the pendulum doesn't seem to work. Gradually you will learn how to find the information another way or to do what is necessary to avoid the problems. I've been keeping a list of such problems for several months, and it's gotten long. These are all situations that you need to know about, and what to do if you encounter them.

Almost everything on the list below can be avoided or corrected. Most of the answers come with experience, with using pendulums enough to learn the fine points of how to ask questions and receive answers, and with learning how to use the tool itself. A number of these problems have already been discussed, but this chapter brings them all together in one place. Though a pendulum works like a computer, it is much simpler, and so are the difficulties that you will face in using it. I have numbered the items covered here for easier use, to make the material readily available when you need it.

If you continue to have difficulty working with your pendulum and achieving accurate, useful information from it, one suggestion is to take your difficulty to the Light-being who is running it with you. Ask for her help. With a series of pendulum questions, she may be able to convey to you what you need to do to resolve the problem. She may also be able to take care of it from her end. If this doesn't work, you might take your request for help to the Lords of Karma—the way to do this is the subject of chapter eleven.

Another suggestion is to reread the instructions covered in this book. Something you have missed or decided not to do could be the source of your difficulty. Everything in this book is suggested because I know it is important and it works. If you are not keeping your pendulums absolutely energetically cleared, for example, or have not dedicated them or yourself to the Light—there is your problem without having to look further. If you observe the information in this book, you should be able to achieve 95 percent accuracy with your pendulum for most types of requests, including for psychic readings. Even when asking about the future, you should be able to achieve about 75 percent accuracy.

As you become more experienced with pendulum use, you may find other situations to add to the following list. You will also find your own answers for resolving the situations. Nothing is ever the last word or final information on any subject, and I cannot pretend that this book is the final word either. There is always something more to learn. The purpose of this book is to get you started. Once you have learned the teaching here, you will go further on your own, and you will have the means and background to be able to do so. If you continue beyond the teachings of this book, I've done my job and you are doing yours.

1. First on the list is *poor focus and concentration.* To be able to attain accurate pendulum responses and information, you need to focus your mind at all times on the question you are asking.

   Pendulum use is a mental process, involving the mind (which is more than the brain) and how you think and use your power of thought. Thought transmission is fragile. Your thought is how you speak to your Be-ing of the Highest Light and how you ask your questions. You think them. When that thought communication reaches your Light-being, her response is transmitted through you to register in the swinging weight on a chain that is your pendulum.

The response doesn't move directly from your Light-being to the pendulum. It has to be transmitted through your subconscious mind and neuromuscular system, which then causes your hand to move the pendulum (however imperceptibly).

This is all a very fragile process, subject to static and interference every step of the way. The primary means of reducing the static is to keep your mind clear and focused on what you are asking. Think your question and keep it in your mind—and nothing else in your mind—until your pendulum registers a response and you understand what the response is.

Poor focus is something you can correct; focusing correctly is a skill that you can learn. If this is something you have had difficulty with in other aspects of your daily life, the pendulum can be your means of healing it. Not only will your pendulum work improve, but so will your ability to concentrate in other ways. For someone with attention deficit disorder, for example, learning to master pendulum use could be one means to greater healing and change. If your concentration with the pendulum is poor for other reasons, you will again find benefit in your life by using the pendulum to learn to focus.

2. Another reason your pendulum might not work properly is that you are allowing yourself to be *distracted*. This might be another aspect of having to learn better focusing skills, but it can also pertain to your working conditions. Until you have developed an unshakable focus and automatic altered state (which not everyone will do), you need to do your pendulum work alone in a quiet place. Especially in the beginning, trying to ask questions with a pendulum in a crowded room, with people moving in and out and other activity going on, can be impossible. Instead of your

mind focusing on the pendulum, you are tuning into the conversation that the other people nearby are having.

However much you may try in a situation like this, your mind will not remain focused. You shouldn't expect it to. Take your pendulum to a quiet room where you can be alone. Close the door, shut off the television, and turn off the phone ringer. Take a few minutes to get centered and to clear your mind. Do some deep breathing. Then try to use your pendulum again. You will have much better results.

If your mind is too distracted, if you have worries that won't wait, you will need to clear the worries before your pendulum will work. Try some of the meditation techniques in chapter five. Look at each worry briefly—don't get hung up on any of them—then let them go. Burn them up in your candle flame, or put them in a magick box or bag to take them out later (if you must take them out at all). In South America, people tell their worries at bedtime to little cloth dolls made for the purpose. Once the worries are given to the dolls, the dolls will take care of them and hopefully find their resolutions. These dolls are available very cheaply in import stores. You might wish to invest in some and use them. You can also designate a teddy bear for the purpose. Keep the doll or bear by your bed and use it. Once you give away your worries, let them go. Try not to take them back again—ever.

With practice, you will learn to put all other concerns and thoughts aside when you pick up your pendulum. The only thoughts to allow in your mind at this time are the questions you are asking, and those only one at a time. By doing your pendulum work in a quiet place, you are on your way to correcting the problem. If you really want to solve the issue of distraction, however, learning to meditate is your long-term answer.

3. Another reason your pendulum gives you wrong answers or doesn't respond at all is because *you are not looking at it.* Looking

at your pendulum is a means of focusing your mind and keeping it focused on the work that you are doing. Watch the weighted end, observing how the pendulum swings. Is it saying "yes" or "no"? Without looking at it, you may find that the pendulum swings wildly. Once you are very experienced and proficient with the pendulum, you may not need to do this, but the time for that has yet to come.

If you are making a request about an object, you can look at the object rather than at your pendulum. For example, if you are asking which of two cucumbers to buy in the supermarket, look at the first one and ask, "Is this the best cucumber for me to buy?" When you ask the same question about the other one, change your visual focus to look at the second one, in turn. Vision is the origin of your short-term memory, and it is one of the origins of your ability to focus your mind.

4. If you are not proficient in understanding the pendulum's responses—if you *don't recognize "yes," "no," and "maybe"*—you will not be able to use the pendulum at all. Everything you need in order to learn this is in chapter six. Read it if you haven't already, or read it again and go through the exercises. If you need to, repeat the exercises daily until you immediately and automatically know your pendulum's communication code—how it will swing to tell you "yes," "no," and "maybe."

Ask your Be-ing of the Highest Light to help you with every step and to help you to resolve your difficulties. Once you have learned to work with the Lords of Karma, you may ask for their help as well. Don't expect your pendulum to actually "talk" to you and don't expect the responses to be large. These are quiet, subtle reactions. Watch the weight of the pendulum move on the end of the chain. That's the response you are looking for.

5. One of the most frequent reasons pendulums don't work accurately is that they are *not kept absolutely energetically cleared at all*

times. The thought transmission that pendulum work is based upon is a fragile form of electrical energy. Electricity attracts static, which then interferes with the reception. Clearing your pendulum removes the static, making communication possible again. A pendulum in need of cleansing is never accurate and may not work at all; it might swing in meaningless circles. It can even swing wildly enough to fly out of your hand and break.

Your pendulums should be cleared before their first use and after every use, and they should be kept in the cleansing medium whenever they are not in your hand. You should use a pendulum for no more than two hours before switching to a purified one or before cleansing the one you've been using before continuing with it. The quickest and simplest method of pendulum cleansing is to place in it a small bowl of water to which a handful of dry sea salt has been added. Let the pendulum soak in the salt water for at least half an hour, or until when you ask, "Is this pendulum absolutely energetically cleared?" you get a "yes." Never use a pendulum that is not completely cleared, or at least cleared enough for your Light-being to say that you can still work with it. Working with an uncleared pendulum is a waste of time. Your responses will never be accurate or useful.

6. A crucial reason pendulums are unreliable is when *they are not being run by a Be-ing of the Highest Light.* In order for the connection with a Light-being to happen, you first must dedicate yourself to the Light. This states your clear intent and establishes which side you are on, so to speak. If you are not on the side of the Light, you are not a safe energy for a Light-being to work through. A Be-ing of the Highest Light will not work for evil, and there is no neutral or in-between here—you are either of the Light or you are not.

    This dedication is not in violation of any religion, other than perhaps Satanism (which *is* evil). Dedication is the primary means of initiating evolution and protection for you. It also protects any Be-ing of the Light that might choose to work with you. No Be-ing of the Highest Light will run your pendulum, help you, teach you, or provide you with information if you are not dedicated to the Light. Unless your choice is to be evil, there is no reason to refuse to dedicate yourself.

Once you have dedicated yourself to the Light and develop a relationship with a Light-being, your pendulum will be more accurate and reliable than it ever could have been before. Look over chapter four, on dedication, again. You only have to say aloud three times, "I dedicate myself and my life, and all my lifetimes and between them, to the Light" for it to be so. If you have done the dedication, your connection to the Light and Light-being guidance is there, and it will never leave you again.

7. You also will not make connection with a Light-being, or your Light-being will not work with or for you, if *you treat your Be-ing of the Highest Light with anything less than total respect.* This is probably a very rare occurrence, but it happens. There are a few immature people who have no gratitude or understanding of the blessings they are being offered. If this is you, change your attitude immediately. Otherwise, you may someday regret what it will cost you.

8. If you use your pendulum to *ask trivial questions, you will get trivial responses.* Likewise, if you ask questions that you don't really want to know, don't need to know, or that it isn't for your highest good to know, you will not receive valid answers. No questions that violate the privacy or free will of others will be answered, nor will questions about other people if you have no right to know the information. When you separate your ego and pride from your desire to use the pendulum, and you enter into a path of spiritual evolution, you will be given all the answers that you need. When you enter into a path of service to others, to the Earth, or to the

Light, you will be given a course of higher instruction and more information than you could ever imagine having.

The pendulum is not a toy or a parlor game. It is a serious tool for serious learning and psychic work. Respect it as such, and you will gain greatly from it. Disrespect it and it will give you nothing.

9. *Poor phrasing of your questions* can make your pendulum responses garbled and meaningless. To use a pendulum, you need to ask extremely simple questions with extremely simple "yes" or "no" answers. If your question contains the words "and" or "or," you will need to separate it into two different queries. Ask only one question at a time. Use phrasing and wording that is totally unambiguous (that can only mean one thing). Use the most precise wording that you can, and ask for exactly what you wish to know.

    Pendulum use is the art of asking questions that can give you the most clear information with a limited range of responses. It's a skill that takes some time to develop. Experiment with it, and keep using the pendulum, and with practice you will get the knack. Every chapter in this book has examples of how to ask questions with a pendulum.

10. *Doubt* can interfere with your pendulum use by making you think, "I can't do it" or "This isn't worth doing." What you think is what you create. The questions here are, Do you want to use a pendulum for information and spiritual evolution? Do you want to work with a Light-being who will guide your growth? If so, then stop allowing any interference. Such interference may come in the form of doubting parents, housemates, or friends. (Is such a person really your friend?) It can also come from trying to perform, to show others who may not be open to what you can do. The skeptics don't need to know, and you don't need to waste your time convincing them. Their growth is at risk; don't let them jeopardize yours.

Such people who implant doubt in your mind or cause you to waver on your path are not Light-beings. They are ignorant, negative, and destructive—and may even be evil. Your job in this is to be the best that you can be, and that means to reject doubt and those who make you doubt, and go forward with your evolution and growth. This might not be easy, but I did it, and so can you.

11. Interference can also be from *discarnate entities that are not of the Light*. These can be attachments, negative elementals, negative spirits, and other negative or evil entities and Be-ings. Evil is real and it exists. We encounter it every day. Entities can manipulate your thinking or your pendulum. If your thoughts are negative, they may have been manipulated. We are all under attack, and if you are just starting on a path of Light, you are especially vulnerable.

What to do? First dedicate yourself to the Light; then start asking for protection and for help. You will not be refused. Reject all that you know is not positive and good. Refuse all negative or evil thoughts and all thoughts of destruction for yourself and all others. Ask daily, as many times as you can, to be "filled with so much Light that nothing that is not the Light can enter, remain, or harm me."

Dedicate your pendulums to the Light and keep them absolutely energetically cleared at all times. If your pendulum swings in such a way that all your answers are "no," ask if a Be-ing of the Light is running your pendulum. If it is not, demand that the entity leave and never return. Ask for the help of Archangel Michael or any other Protector of the Light. Ask him to destroy the entity if it is evil or to take it to where it belongs if it is not evil. Never allow evil to run your pendulums or to communicate with you. Once the entity has gone, place the pendulum in dry sea salt and leave it there for a week. You will probably have to destroy the pendulum. Even if the entity has left, it is likely that the pendulum will no longer be alive. All of this is very serious, and you must take it seriously. Reject all that is negative and evil, and ask for the protection of the Light—now, forever, and always.

12. Your pendulum will not work in any meaningful way if you run it while experiencing any type of *negative emotional state*. This means that you cannot depend on the accuracy of your pendulum if you run it while you are angry, terrified, or upset. It may not run accurately if you are ill. During a time of trauma and crisis or of extreme exhaustion, your pendulum may not operate effectively either. Your pendulum works through the medium of your mind, and your mind is definitely influenced by emotion. To use a pendulum effectively, you must focus and clear your mind, and your emotions must be neutral. If they are not, they will influence your responses, and your pendulums may simply swing wildly, giving you no response at all. Even if you think that your pendulum is working during times of high emotion, be very careful about depending upon its information. It probably will not be accurate until you can calm down and regain your neutrality and your focus.

13. Likewise, if you *want a particular response very badly,* your pendulum can give it to you. This is not what you want from a guidance tool, however—what you really want is truth. This is another situation where you can't depend upon accurate responses because your emotions will interfere with the guidance. To prevent this interference, you must learn to keep your mind focused and your emotions neutral. It's a skill that you can learn. If you want something very badly, ask someone else to question the pendulum about it for you. Your answers, if you do it yourself, won't be the truth. Wishing can swing the pendulum, but it won't make what you desire come to pass.

14. Another occasion when you should not use a pendulum is *when you are under the influence of alcohol or drugs.* Any substance that

negatively affects your mind will affect your pendulum. This includes some prescription drugs, by the way. Any substance that causes change in your inhibitions or judgment will affect your pendulum's responses and reliability. Your Be-ing of the Highest Light will not be able to communicate with you or offer you guidance. The influence of alcohol or drugs can also attract negative entities, which could cause you harm and place your Light-being in danger. You can choose to put yourself at risk, but be aware of the consequences. Don't pick up your pendulum until you are sober, as the responses you get from it will not be useful, and it may have been taken over by an entity that is not of the Light.

15. If you are *obsessed with a situation or overinvolved with a situation, person, or subject,* your pendulum will not be reliable or useful. The effect is similar to both strong emotions and the influence of negative substances—an obsession can be an addiction that operates in your thinking like alcohol or a drug. In both of these cases, your mind cannot be focused or your emotions made neutral. Your obsession or overinvolvement will infiltrate your thinking and influence every response to every question you may ask. The first part of your healing is to recognize that your thinking is not in your highest good. The second part is to seek help, whether that be from therapy, a 12-step program, or breaking off contact with the situation or person involved. Once you let go, close the door and don't open it again.

Your pendulum and your Be-ing of the Highest Light cannot help you if you will not help yourself. Pendulum use depends on a clear and focused mind, not a mind stuck on a subject and unable to break free or to think of anything else. There may be attachments or entities that are not of the Light involved. Dedicate yourself to the Light and ask for help. You will not be refused, but you must also be willing to do everything you can for yourself.

Use the guidance you receive from your pendulum and your Be-ing of the Highest Light to heal yourself.

16. Your pendulum will not be accurate if *you ask the same request over and over again.* If you know that a Be-ing of the Highest Light is operating your energetically cleared pendulum, and your mind is focused and your emotions are neutral when you make your request, accept the answer you are given. Your Light-being will give you truth, and only truth, but you must be willing to hear it. If the answer is not what you wanted, repeating the question will not change it. You can influence the pendulum and change the answer for yourself if you want to, but how will that serve? Do you want truth or wishful thinking? The choice is up to you.

    If you have been given an answer to your question, don't ask again unless you have reason to believe that something has changed in the situation. You can ask your pendulum if that is the case. If something has changed, and you are told that it has, you may want to repeat your query. Usually, however, your first answer is the real one and you do best by accepting it. Don't ask your question any more often than is reasonable, and what is reasonable can vary with the situation. Trust your Be-ing of the Highest Light.

17. *Lack of common sense* can get anyone into any amount of trouble, and this is true with pendulums as well. Never accept an answer from the pendulum that you know to be untrue. Never act upon pendulum information that will cause you or anyone else harm of any kind. Any information that tells you to do something neg-ative, evil, or against your highest good (or anyone else's) is to be ignored—it is not of the Light. If you receive information through your pendulum that you can't readily accept, do what you can to verify it. Never do anything that you know to be eth-ically wrong, no matter who tells you (or who you think is telling you) to do it.

Always ask before you begin using your pendulum, "Is a Be-ing of the Highest Light running this pendulum?" If not, accept that nothing you are given is the truth. Never use a pendulum that is not absolutely energetically cleared and being run by a Light-being. If your Be-ing of the Highest Light is truly running your pendulum, however, the information in question may be correct. You can wait to make sure before you act, and the Light will applaud you for your caution. Accept only the truth, and do your best to find out what the truth is. The truth will always be a factor of your common sense.

18. Your pendulum will not give you useful information if *your thoughts contradict themselves or if you keep changing your mind.* This is when what you decide is true when you start to ask the question shifts while you are asking it, and it shifts again a moment after that. The pendulum reflects your changing mind, saying "yes" and then "no" to the same changing question. No one can keep up with your indecisiveness, not even the Be-ing of the Light that is attempting to guide you. This is another case where you need to calm yourself and learn to focus your mind. If you can keep your mind still and steady, your eyes on the pendulum, and can hold one thought the whole time you are asking the question, you may have a chance for some guidance that will resolve your situation. Do your best to give that guidance a chance.

Again, here is where meditation techniques of putting your worries away or on hold would help you greatly. Try the South American worry dolls or the worry bear. If you can't make a clear decision, maybe you need more information. Try to refrain from vacillating until you have the information that might show you a clearer path. If you keep contradicting yourself, you will only become more confused. Maybe you need to have a talk with someone whose wisdom and common sense you respect and leave the pendulum alone until you do. Once you know what to think, and can make up your mind and stay with it, you might be able to use your pendulum's advice again.

Sometimes your own mind is made up, and the pendulum responses still vacillate and contradict. The responses may be so contradictory that you may wonder if there is a negative entity running your pendulum, but you are assured that there is not. In this case it is another person involved who can't make up *her* mind. Sometimes this situation comes up when you are using the pendulum to find someone, a person or a pet who is missing or whose whereabouts are unknown. You may get the contradictory responses if the person or animal doesn't want to be found, or can't decide whether or not to come home.

19. Your pendulum may not give you the information you are asking for if *you are not open to receive the information or the Light-being that offers it, or if you are very afraid of the answer.* In this case, you may not believe that the Be-ing running the pendulum with you is truly of the Light, or you may be afraid of being judged or punished (two things that no one of the Light will do). You may not trust a Be-ing of the Light because you do not know what that means. You may have been raised in a religion that has taught you to be afraid. If you can't accept the source of your information, you will be wary of the information itself and be afraid to trust both the information and the bearer.

You may also be afraid of the answer to your question and not sure that you really want to know. If you have ever had to ask your pendulum and Light-being such questions as, "Am I dying?" or "Do I have cancer?" or "Is my mother about to die?" your fear is understandable.

Probably the issue here is trust and truth. You must decide to trust the Light. If it is a Be-ing of the Highest Light running your pendulum, clear your mind and your fears, and let her help you.

20. One reason you may have difficulty in determining your pendulum's responses is that *you are working too fast,* and your pendulum doesn't have the time to clear itself from one response before it goes into the next. This is why you need to watch your pendulum while you are asking for answers. By doing this, you will prevent yourself from asking another question before you receive the response to the first. I use my pendulums very rapidly; others who work with me can't keep up. I work too fast even for myself sometimes, and occasionally I get ahead of myself. The pendulum at that point just swings, usually in an exaggerated "yes," until I slow down and ask the questions again. Sometimes at such high speeds, however, the responses are just delayed, but they come in the sequence in which I asked the questions. I see a series of responses for which I might no longer remember the questions! As with a lot of things, do as I say and not as I do. Slow down! That's all it takes to solve the problem. You may have to ask a couple of your questions over again to understand the answers.

21. *Using the pendulum for prophecy* when you're not proficient enough in it, or when your Be-ing of the Highest Light is not willing to aid you, will cause unreliable and inaccurate responses. If your Light-being refuses to do such future requests with you, it is usually because she feels you are not ready to do this advanced work. Your ability to phrase questions has to be very precise for future work to have value. You need to understand that what may be predictable (or predicted) today could change totally tomorrow, when someone makes a different decision or changes their mind. You also need to be aware that your accuracy will be less with future work than with any other aspect of using pendulums.

Prophecy and inquiries into the future involve multiple possibilities and realities. The information you receive can be one of many alternatives. As decisions are made and minds change and events happen, the possibilities and probabilities shift. What looked like the best possibility yesterday may not be so today, and tomorrow something else entirely could manifest. The Lords of Karma tell us to heal the past and the present, and the future will take care of itself. It may be best to worry about tomorrow when it comes, but most of us still want to know. Do future work only for yourself, and be aware of the limitations of the information you receive.

22. Your pendulum will not be accurate or provide useful guidance when you *gamble*. Don't expect help from your pendulum or your Be-ing of the Highest Light in any form of this endeavor. They will not help you pick lottery numbers, racing wins, or even manifest for you that last spot you need to win at Bingo. In my understanding of this, it is the Light that chooses the winners, not us—and we are not to be involved. Gambling, as a whole, is frowned upon by the Light.

23. Until you are connected with a Be-ing of the Light, *fluorescent lighting* may interfere with the accuracy and function of your pendulum. Once you are connected with a Light-being, this effect seems to lessen or disappear. I don't know why this form of lighting affects pendulums or why dedication to the Light stops the interference. I only know that it is so.

24. *Heavy lightning during thunderstorms* or the low barometric pressure that goes with thunderstorms and severe weather can affect pendulum use. In my experience, it seems that the pendulum will register an exaggerated "yes" and not respond in any other way until the worst of the storm is over. My guessed explanation for this is that lightning is an electrical energy that interferes with the delicate electricity of thought transmission.

25. This last reason for why your pendulums aren't working properly should be a no-brainer: *if you are not working for the Light, or in accordance with the Light in all requests, do not expect help from your pendulum.* This doesn't even need an explanation.

This should cover most of the reasons a pendulum does not give you the clear information that you think it should. This list may not cover all the situations that could ever occur, but it should be enough to give you what you need. Use the troubleshooting information to make your pendulum use more reliable in every way that you can.

USING CHARTS

Some people who work with pendulums like to use charts, maps, and lists with them. Doing this increases the amount of information you can receive because it enables the pendulum to choose from a selection of possibilities. This might mean the pendulum picking (swinging "yes") to indicate one item from a list of several or many items, to indicate a specific place on a map or anatomy chart, or to indicate one of a variety of other concepts or words. Pendulum charts can be circular or fan shaped, written columns or lists of words or ideas, anatomical charts, number or letter increments, rows of pictures, or maps of anything, from the world to your living room.

Traditional dowsers use pendulums and dowsing tools to locate water, geopathic zones, minerals, metals, lost people, or lost objects, and they find what they seek by using charts and maps. With these aids, they determine where to search without having to go there physically or walk over miles of terrain while waiting for their dowsing tools to respond. They first narrow their search to where the pendulum or dowser indicates "yes" on the map. Next they go in person to a much smaller and more contained area than would have been possible to do otherwise, where they then complete the search. Doing it this way, they find what they seek more quickly and easily. Such techniques are similar to doing distance healing and are called *teleradiesthesia*.

This manner of traditional dowsing, though often considered old-fashioned by today's New Age pendulum users, works very well. It is not a method to let slip into disuse but to teach to newer generations. While there is less need today to locate where to dig a well for drinking water, and mining is done by high technology, these techniques still work. They have a great many valid and important applications and can be expanded to a great many uses. Like most pendulum work, their uses can be applied to your every need and are only limited by your imagination. They are an important aspect of using the pendulum as an information tool.

Working with maps and charts expands your pendulum choices and increases the yes-no (and maybe) pendulum vocabulary considerably. It adds greatly to the pendulum binary code by adding "which one" (or "which one of many choices") to your list of possible answers. Instead of holding a vitamin in your hand and asking, "Is this something I need?" you run your finger slowly over a list of many vitamins, minerals, and supplements and ask, "Which of all of these do I need?" When your finger touches something appropriate, the pendulum swings to "yes." It swings to "yes" for everything on the list that you need, whether that means one vitamin or ten. Instead of asking about each item, one by one, you ask about them as a group. This gives you much more information in much less time.

For a simple way to begin this, try the following. You are ready to buy a new car and you have several choices. You want to know which of four cars would be the best for you to buy. All of them are within your price range, all of them have a reasonable service reputation, and you like them all. They are approximately equal, as far as you are aware, but you can only buy one, so which is it to be? As you've used your pendulum so far, you can touch each of the four cars, one by one, with your non-dominant hand, while holding your pendulum in your dominant hand. Then, with each car, ask your Be-ing of the Highest Light, "Is this the car I should buy?" Once you have tried this with all four cars, you will have your answer.

To simplify this, you might instead hold Car A in your mind and think of it while asking with the pendulum, "Should I buy Car A?" You would do this with each of the four cars and again find your answer. Sometimes in a situation like this, where all choices are equal, your pendulum can actually swing "yes" for all four choices. Then it's up to you to decide, though it's rare for all the choices in any situation to be equal. To simplify it further, you might write the description of each car on four identical small pieces of paper. Car A is a Mazda, so write "Mazda" on the paper; car B is a Chevy, so write "Chevy" on another piece of paper; and so on, for cars C and D. Turn the pieces of paper face down and mix them up so you don't see the names; you're letting the Light pick for you.

Now take your pendulum and hold it over the first piece of paper and ask, "Is this the car I should buy?" "No." Hold it over the second piece of paper and ask, "Is this the car I should buy?" "No." Do it the third time, and this is your "yes." Turn the paper over, and you have your choice. Verify it in your own mind before buying it, and be sure that this is truly the car you want—it's an expensive purchase. Another way to do this is to ask the question, "Which of these cars should I buy?" Hold your pendulum over the four pieces of paper that are face down. It will register "yes" when you hold it over the best choice, and show you "no" over all the other pieces. In this case, you have asked your question only once and gotten four responses (one of which is "yes" and your new car).

In another beginning way of using charts and lists, cut pictures of each of the four cars from a magazine and spread them out in front of you on a table. Holding your pendulum in your dominant hand, ask your Be-ing of the Highest Light, "Which of these cars is best for me to buy?" Hold the question in your mind, but keep your mind clear of thinking about any of the cars, and stay emotionally neutral. (If you have an emotion about one of the cars, that car is what your pendulum will pick.) With the question in your mind, hold your pendulum over the pictures one at a time. Give your pendulum time to react to each, and look at each picture as your pendulum hangs over it. When you are over the picture of the optimal car, your pendulum will swing to "yes."

In the last examples, you asked about choices you could not look at, and then you asked about choices you could see. The names of the cars on pieces of paper were face down, so you couldn't see them; the photos of the cars were face up, so you could. Which method gave you better information or a clearer choice? Did both of the methods tell you to buy the same car? In the example of the car, you had four choices, and your graphics (the pieces of paper and the pictures) were quite simple. Such graphic aids can be simple or complicated, and they can contain any number of choices or items to choose from.

Try the above methods to predict something that will happen shortly in the future. It is best to avoid gambling questions, as you will not get a valid response, but try something else, such as, which one of four people being interviewed will your boss hire? In this case, you would write their names on four small identical pieces of paper, put the papers face down, and ask your pendulum to show you who will be hired. Make your request as you did above. Hold your pendulum over each piece of paper in turn, not moving it to the next piece until you have a response. When you get the "yes," turn over the paper and see who is coming to work with you. If the hiring were actually under way, you would soon be able to verify the accuracy of your pendulum's information.

Then do the second part of the exercise. You probably wouldn't have photographs of the candidates, but you might have their applications. Hold your pendulum over each application, making the same request as you did before. Do you get the same response or not? Is it possible that person A (that your pendulum said "yes" to before) was offered the job and refused it, and that person B (who got the "yes" when the pendulum was held over the applications) is the person actually coming to work? Remember that prophecy can be tricky that way. Person A may have been offered the job, as your pendulum indicated, but she didn't accept the offer. Your pendulum may indicate that you should buy car B, but your own inclination is to buy car A. When you get to the store, however, car A has been sold—and you come home with car B after all. Be aware of how things change and how they work out when you are using a psychic tool. Some of the "coincidences" will surprise you.

To expand your use of these multiple-choice pendulum aids and to give you many more choices, try using lists. Before we discuss them, however, I need to state that the lists and charts described and shown in this book are only examples to get you started. You can make your own lists, charts, and maps that are tailored to whatever purposes you need. There also are dozens of books of pendulum charts on the market, some of them beautifully designed. New ones seem to come out every day. While many of these are interesting and they can be highly useful, I find it much more useful to make my own. That way, all of the items or choices that I wish to list are included, without extraneous things that I don't want or need. To be useful, charts and lists only need to include the choices you require; it doesn't matter where they come from or whether or not they were professionally made.

To give you an idea of how to use a list, consider the example that follows. You are using the telephone directory to find a plumber. There are dozens of plumbers listed for your area, and you want to know several things before you pick one to call. You don't know any of these plumbers and have never used any of their services. In your mind they are all equal because they are all unknown. You need the name of only one, but that one must meet the following criteria: he or she must do good work that he or she is willing to guarantee, do it at the lowest possible cost, be reliable, and be someone you feel safe having in your home. Clearing your mind of everything else, you state your criteria clearly to your Be-ing of the Highest Light and ask her to choose which plumber to call.

Now, pick up your absolutely energetically cleared pendulum. Hold it over the opened phone directory, where there are several pages of plumbers. Ask your Light-being to show you a "yes" to indicate the page where your best-choice plumber is listed. Hold your pendulum in your right hand (if you are right-handed) and place your opposite hand palm down on the first page. You can also point to the page or touch it with your index finger. Look at the page, asking, "Is the plumber we need listed on this page?" The answer is "no." Go to the next page and do the same. Your plumber, it turns out, is on the third page.

Go to that page, which has four columns of listings for plumbers, and ask your Light-being, "Is my plumber listed in column one? "Yes." Then ask, "Is my plumber listed in the top half of column one on this page?" "No." "Is my plumber listed in the bottom half of column one on this page?" The response is "yes." Place your finger (or use a pencil for a pointer) on the first listing of the lower half of column one. Ask, "Is this my plumber?" "No." Do the same for each listing until you get the "yes." You can also run your pointer down the listings, very slowly, asking your Be-ing of the Highest Light to show you a "yes" when you reach the plumber she has chosen for you. When you get the "yes," verify it by ask-ing, "Is this the best plumber for me to call, one who meets my criteria?" If the answer is "yes," make the call.

I have used this method with great success many times. Be careful not to move your finger or pointer down the list too quickly, as it may pre-vent you from seeing the swing change to "yes." Your pendulum will swing in a slow "no" response until you indicate the correct page, col-umn, column half, and listing. Then with each correct choice the swing will change. A telephone book contains a dense amount of information, and the print is very small. Using something as a pointer or indicator will help you, as your finger can cover several listings at once. A pen or pen-cil works fine for this.

You can try this with want ads, shopping ads, lists of herbs or gem-stones, names of doctors, chiropractors, handymen—virtually anything. You can choose from lists of books or entrées on a menu; you can ask, "Which book?" "Which dinner?" "Which dessert?" I have a food allergy to bell peppers, and it is always aggravating to order in restaurants. Waiters generally don't know or care whether a dish contains peppers or not, and the cooks and chefs refuse to remove them if they do. Sometimes I'm told there are no peppers in the dish, then spend the next few days being ill from them. I use my pendulum to ask if an entrée that looks interesting has peppers in it. If so, before I attempt asking the waiter or waitress about removing them, I ask the pendulum if they would actually do so. It may not be worth the effort to ask. Instead, I often ask Brede to "Pick me the best dinner," and She always does. She would much rather pick desserts, of course, and they have to be heavy on the chocolate.

For a simple chart to use in finding things, make a floor plan of your house or apartment. (See my example in diagram 2.) It doesn't have to be fancy, but it should diagram each room, as well as your garage, patio, and porches (if you have them), and your yard. Label the rooms. In an earlier example, I talked about finding lost objects and a lost kitten. This time, instead of asking repeated questions like, "Are my keys in the living room?" "Are my keys in the bedroom?" "Are my keys in the garage?" try using the house plan. To do this, with the house chart in front of you and your cleared pendulum held over it, ask of your Light-being, "Show me where to find my missing keys."

There are a couple of ways that you can proceed from this point. As you did with choosing a plumber, you can use your finger or a pointer to point to each room of your house, represented on the house plan chart. Look at each room one by one. Place your pointer or finger on the square that represents each room, focusing on one room at a time. Work slowly, allowing your pendulum to register a response before moving on. Your pendulum will swing "no" until you touch the room where your keys are. Then the swing will shift to "yes." Before beginning this, you might ask with your pendulum, "Are my keys in the house?" They might not be. "Are they outdoors?" "Are they in the yard?" "Did I drop them on the porch?" are all possible questions. If these are included in your house plan chart, you won't need to ask separate questions; the locations will already be on the map.

Try using your pendulum in a different way. This time with the chart facing toward you, hold your pendulum motionless at the center lower edge of the house plan. On my chart, this is where the lower edge of the

DIAGRAM 2
HOUSE PLAN CHART

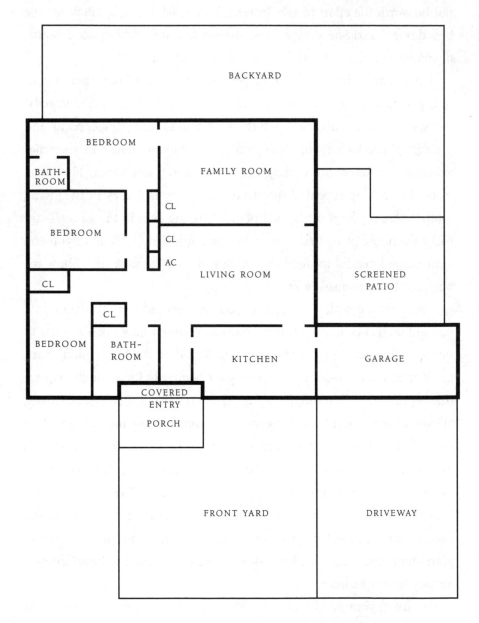

Make a floor plan of your house or apartment to use as a chart to find things. The chart's hinge point is at the lower edge of the diagram; in this case, where the front yard and driveway meet.

front yard and driveway meet. On other houses, it might be before the front door. This center point on a pendulum chart is called "the hinge." Ask your Be-ing of the Highest Light, "Show me where to find my missing keys." Look at your pendulum and keep your mind empty. The pendulum will slowly begin to swing, and the weighted end will pull in the direction (or actually go to the room on the diagram) where the keys may be found. This is a form of the "yes" response.

It is odd to see a pendulum vary its usual swing to pull the pendant end toward the left or right of the diagram. If it pulls to the left and you are not sure of the room, use your finger or pointer to find *which* room on the left. Ask again, "Show me where to find my missing keys." Or ask, "Which room?" The pendulum will swing "yes" when you touch the correct room, or it will pull to indicate the correct room if you continue to hold it at the "hinge point." Be aware that this is a pendulum skill that may not work for everyone. You can use this pendulum pulling method with most charts or diagrams but not with lists.

In summary, hold your pendulum steady and still at the center of the lower edge of the map or chart, or just below the bottom of the diagram at its center. The position is called "the hinge." Make your request, with your mind clear and your eyes on the pendulum. The way the pendulum pulls will lead you to the information you are asking for. The movement will be quite different from your usual "yes" or "no" swings, but the information is still your "yes."

The next type of chart to try this with is the fan chart. This chart holds any kind of information divided into sections on a half circle. You can have as many sections as you wish, but if they are too close together you will have difficulty in discerning which the pendulum indicates when it pulls toward one of them. You can label this chart in any way, with each section listing a choice. In the example above of which automobile to buy, you could have used a fan chart for the request. In this case the sections might be labeled "Mazda," "Chevy," "Geo," "Toyota," and so on. The "hinge point" where you hold your pendulum to start from is at the place below

DIAGRAM 3

BLANK FAN CHART

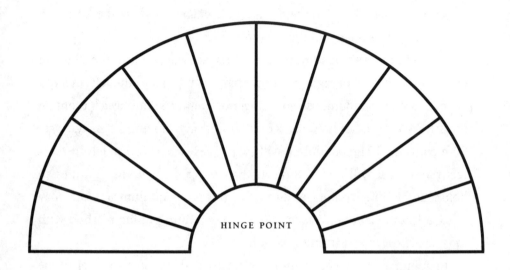

HINGE POINT

You can fill in this chart any way you choose, with each section listing a choice. Hold your pendulum at the hinge point to start. This point is where all the possibilities come together.

Diagram 4

Expanded Response Fan Chart

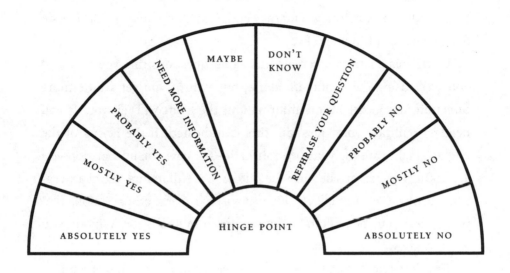

Use this fan chart to expand "yes" and
"no" to ten incremental possibilities.

the center bottom of the fan where all the possibilities come together. Diagrams 3 and 4 show a blank fan chart and one that is filled in.

I have titled the filled-in chart an "Expanded Response Fan Chart." Its sections are incremental gradations of "yes" and "no," to give you more information with your pendulum than the usual binary code. The choices begin with "Absolutely yes," and they end with "Absolutely no." There are five gradations of "no" and five of "yes."

Using this chart, you can ask the same questions that you would if you were using the pendulum alone, but with it you get a little more direction. If you need more information, the chart will tell you. If you need to rephrase your question, this is indicated. If the Be-ing of the Highest Light running your pendulum doesn't have the information you are asking for, perhaps because the outcome is still in flux, the chart registers it with "Don't know." It might be useful to add other sections that read "Clear your pendulum," "Not supposed to know," or "Why do you want to know?"

Fan charts can be drawn for any purpose. If your question is about percentages, amounts, or quantities, they can be divided into increments of numbers. Always make your progression a sequential one—don't skip around. For example, if your chart is about percentages, start at the left with 100 percent and end at the right with 0. The numbers designated in the sections between 100 and 0 might be 80 percent, 60 percent, 40 percent, and 20 percent, in that order. Keep them in descending increments. In the typical design of these charts, the highest numbers (or most favorable answer) are usually at the bottom left-hand side, with decreasing values as the numbers (or words) move from left to right. The right bottom of the fan chart is always your least favorable response. The "hinge point" is always at the center.

Use fan charts for choosing increments of color for color therapy or decorating; the chakra spectrum starts with violet and ends with red. Fan chart divisions can each contain a choice of herb, gemstone, homeopathic remedy, vitamin, or supplement. Such charts are easily designed

for healing uses (see chapter ten). Since fan charts can be adapted for virtually any series of questions that encompasses a small number of possibilities or choices, there are endless ways to use them.

After the fan, or half-circle, chart, try a full circle or wheel. In this type
of pendulum chart, the "hinge point" is at the exact center, in the middle
of the chart. The information possibilities surround the "hinge point."
Probably the easiest example of one of these to imagine is a clock face. (See
diagram 5.) This chart is generally used for questions about time, though
like the fan chart you can designate the increments to mean anything you
wish. The basic chart looks like a clock without hands, numbered as
clocks normally are. You can use a twelve-hour or twenty-four-hour clock.

If you use a twelve-hour clock, you will sometimes need to ask
whether your answer about time is in the A.M. or P.M., and this might be
your first question. You can do this with a horizontal line drawn at the
bottom below the clock. One end of the line says A.M. and the other P.M.
To determine which it is, hold your pendulum over the line, asking,
"When will Lucy get home, A.M. or P.M.?" The pendulum will pull toward
the correct answer. If it does not do this, designate A.M. as "yes" and P.M.
as "no." Tell your Light-being that this is the code you will use with this
chart. A "yes" or "no" from the pendulum will then give you A.M. or P.M.

When the pendulum is held over the number of the hour when Lucy
will arrive, it swings to "yes." To determine the minutes, designate that you
are asking for minutes, and hold the pendulum over the clock numbers.
You will get your "yes" at the correct minutes after the hour. Remember
that time questions can be difficult for a Be-ing of the Highest Light. Some
can do it and some can't seem to give you reliable information. Whatever
time you are given, it may be close, but probably it will not be exact.

Use similar circle or wheel charts for other information using time
requests. Make them to reflect the Wiccan Wheel of the Year, listing the
seasons and Sabbats. Make a circle chart that is a Moon Wheel, a month
calendar with moon phase increments. This type of chart can be used for
the signs and dates of the zodiac. Such charts can be used for "when"

DIAGRAM 5

CLOCK CHART

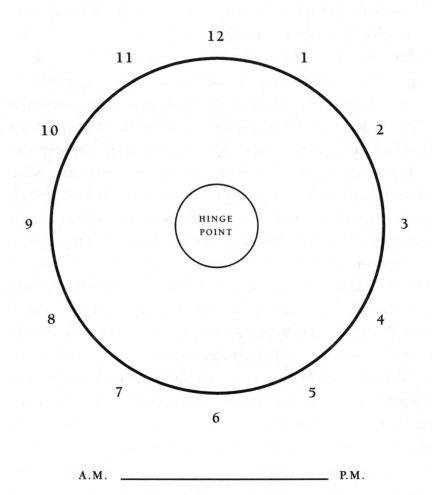

As with the fan chart, you can designate the increments to mean anything you wish, but this chart is usually used for determining time. You can use a twelve- or twenty-four-hour clock.

questions, as in what sign or month or moon phase did (or will) an event you want to know about happen? "Show me the zodiac sign of my cat." "When is the best date to start my vacation?" "What phase of the moon are we in tonight?" "What would be the best date to hold a party or a ritual?" Make a full-circle chart with calendar instead of clock increments to use in questions about dates or days of the standard or lunar calendar month.

You can also make a full-circle chart into something like a Ouija board—a popular game that asks discarnate entities to pull a disk back and forth across an alphabet board, spelling out messages. These are in the "don't touch it with a ten-foot pole" department, as most of the entities that are drawn to communicate through Ouija boards are low level. Most people also use them less than seriously, drawing negative responses that they don't know how to handle. Once you have been dedicated to the Light, however, as long as you specify and absolutely insist that "only a Be-ing of the Highest Light is permitted to run this tool," you might wish to try it. Make a full-circle or wheel chart, but instead of clock numbers this time, put the letters of the alphabet around the edge of the circle.

Using the center of the alphabet wheel as your "hinge point," ask your Be-ing of the Highest Light if she is willing to write you a message using the chart. Your pendulum will be pulled to each letter. Write the letters down one by one. The letters will spell out words, and you will receive your message, though the process is a bit tedious. If your Light-being chooses not to do this, don't insist. If she won't or can't pull your pendulum to indicate the letters for you, you will have to hold the pendulum over each letter, letter after letter, until you get a "yes" for each letter that makes up each word of your message. You will get your message this way but only very slowly. It is probably best not to use these charts for prophecy or psychic readings. They are tedious to use and not as reliable as you can be when using the pendulum alone.

Perhaps I had better confess at this point that Brede won't use charts with me at all, though She is willing to use the written lists. She is also unwilling to run the pendulum by pulling it to indicate the response, though I have experienced this with other Light-beings. She tells me that She is not *unable* to do these things, but that She doesn't *like* to use a pendulum in these ways. If She is unwilling, possibly other Be-ings of the Highest Light may be unwilling to work this way too. If the Light-being that runs your pendulum is unwilling to do something, honor her and find a different way; never argue, as there will always be a good reason. You will get all the information that you need with other methods.

I have honestly never found a need to use charts. My work with the pendulum alone gives me everything that I could need or possibly want. Many people who use pendulums consider charts their most valuable tools, however, and I could not write a pendulum book without discussing them. I personally feel that anything you can do with a chart you can do as well, or better, with a well-phrased question and a "yes" or "no" response. If you are going to use charts, I suggest that you design your own rather than use others from books, and design them to reflect your individual needs.

I will discuss one more type of chart before closing this chapter. Like the house plan, this will help you to find things. Maps are a primary form of charts used by traditional dowsers. You can use them to find anything in as large an area as the world, or as small an area as your backyard. The general way that this is done is to start with a map of a large area, as large an area as you think you will need. Then as you narrow your search, change the larger area map for smaller and smaller area maps, until you can pinpoint what you are searching for precisely.

If you wanted to use a pendulum to find where someone lives, and you had no idea of where to start, you might begin with a map of the world. Find which continent the person lives on and then which country. Next use a map of the country and use it to locate which city the person is living in. Now with a map of that city, find the neighborhood or street. If you can get a map of the neighborhood, you might be able to locate the exact house that the person you seek is living in.

Be aware, however, that even if you locate the person correctly she might not be in the place you were led to if you went there tomorrow. The pendulum map will locate where she physically is when you do the search, but that might not be where she lives permanently. If she happens to be traveling at the time, your pendulum could trace her to a hotel that she could check out of at any time. If she doesn't wish to be found, your pendulum could lead you on a merry chase. I know someone who used maps and pendulums to follow her daughter on a summer tour of Europe. She was accurate about 75 percent of the time but was better at finding the country and city than at determining her daughter's location any more closely. Maps were considered useful for dowsers seeking water or in mining. These are stationary items, however, which won't move away once found.

This chapter on using charts and maps is a small beginning for those who are interested in using them. If you wish to learn more, I suggest reading books on dowsing and dowsing methods. You might wish to contact the American Society of Dowsers, Inc. The address is P.O. Box 24, Danville, VT 05828, (882) 684-3417 or (888) 711-9538, and the website is www.dowsers.org. The organization offers traditional dowsing tools, resources, a bookstore, conferences, events, a chat room, and a newsletter.

HEALING WITH PENDULUMS

I have always been primarily a healer, and healing is the most frequent use I make of pendulums. There are countless ways that pendulums are useful in any psychic healing situation. They offer information on what may be wrong and what to do about it. They aid in choosing among healing methods and remedies. I use them to ask how long a remedy is to be taken, how much to take and how often, and how long a dis-ease will last. I use them to ask for the source of the dis-ease, whether the medical system is needed, and whether the situation is physical only or if it is also emotional, mental, or spiritual in origin. Pendulums are useful for determining when a healing process is needed, which type (or types) of process is appropriate, and when the healing is complete.

My work as a healer is fully eclectic. I use Reiki, distance healing, laying on of crystals, and a variety of other psychic healing methods, both direct and distant. Along with psychic healing, I use naturopathy—healing with nutrition, vitamins and minerals, food supplements, herbs, and homeopathy. I use crystals and gemstones of every kind, and flower and gemstone essences that I make myself. Most of all, I work with karmic healing, as I've discussed in a number of my books and will discuss in chapter eleven. In all cases, pendulums are involved every step of the way. Healing is where pendulums come into their own as a vital psychic tool.

For those readers who are less experienced in psychic healing, it is important to understand the legalities and ethics. In the case of legalities, you must be very clear in the fact that healing and medicine are very different disciplines. A healer is not a doctor, and she can be put in danger by claiming medical skills for which she is not licensed by the medical system. Doctors hate the word "healing" and have no use for healers. To avoid persecution and prosecution, you must be aware of this and protect yourself. You can never claim the ability to "cure" anyone.

The work that you do cannot involve prescribing anything, even if it is over-the-counter or an herb. It is illegal, unless you are a medical doctor, to diagnose (to tell someone what her dis-ease is). You cannot tell someone that you will make the dis-ease go away, that it will be either "cured" or "healed." In some states, you are not permitted to touch anyone without a massage license; in some states, you are not permitted to do Reiki without a massage license either. You are not permitted to tell someone that they don't need a doctor or medical treatment. If you are public in your work or charge money for it, you need to check the laws of your county and state to see what other restrictions apply.

So with all of that said, what *can* you do without being harassed, fined, or jailed? You can tell people that what you do is a relaxation technique, that it will aid them in stress reduction, or that you are providing information only. You can promise that what you do for them will "help" them (though you cannot promise "cure"). If you only do healing work for yourself, family, and friends, these concerns are probably not an issue. The government has better things to do than to crack down on Mom's herb potion for the flu. If you work more publicly or feel that you need more protection, however, you might decide that you want to go to massage or acupuncture school and be legally licensed as a healer in a medically recognized field.

If this doesn't appeal to you, you can call your work "spiritual counseling," for which you must obtain religious or nondenominational clergy credentials, which are protections for healers in most states. Such credentials are available from many alternative churches, temples, and groups, including Spiritualist churches—Of A Like Mind or the Covenant of the

Goddess (COG) for Wiccans—and a variety of New Age centers and healers' training schools. Inquire about what these certifications involve and cost before you sign up, and check with your local laws as to what protections they provide.

You can obtain a nondenominational minister's ordination from Universal Ministries or the Universal Life Church, Inc. These have no training requirements, are without charge, and can be requested online. There are probably other such certifications and organizations available, so check the Internet. Contact information for the Universal Life Church, Inc. is 2159 S. Sky Tanner Drive, Tucson, AZ 85748; fax (520) 290-9328. The website is www.ulc.org. I recommend this group: it has been certifying ministers for decades, it has a Priestess Certificate, and members are recognized and accepted worldwide. For Universal Ministries ordination, the address is 201 N. Chicago Street, P.O. Box 31, Milford, IL 60953; www.universalministries.com/ordination. Either of these will provide you with ordination credentials and make your "spiritual counseling" legal. These groups offer a variety of other benefits and resources, though their legality varies from state to state.

Now that we've discussed some of the legal requirements, what about ethics? I believe that what happens in a healing is a three-way agreement between the healer, the person or animal receiving the healing, and the Goddess (or your name for the Source or the Light). The first ethic is that you take credit only for your expertise, not for what benefit may happen in the healing—you are only the channel, the bridge between the Light/Goddess and the healing that occurs. As a healer, you are required to be compassionate, nonjudgmental, and emotionally neutral—caring but detached. No matter what you hear, you are to place no blame. No matter what you learn, it is to be kept confidential. As in all other psychic work, you must not violate anyone's free will. If they agree to the healing you propose to do, you may go ahead with it; otherwise you may not. This goes for situations in which you ask the person directly, as well as for distance-healing situations, where you can receive the permission indirectly by asking the person's Higher Self in meditation. (This works for animals as well as people.) If you do not have permission, you will not be helped by the Light in your work, and your pendulum will not be run by the Light. Healing will not prevent those who are at their time of death from passing over, but it will ease their transition. In most cases, you are not to ask when someone will die.

One further thought here. We who are women in a patriarchal culture have always been the healers, midwives, herbalists, and psychics—and we have been persecuted for it, as men have not been. Early on in my quest to learn healing, I was given a promise by Brede and told that the promise extends to all who do healing in this time and culture. The promise is this: there will be no more Inquisitions. We are safe to learn healing and to be healers. Use your common sense with regard to the legalities, obey the ethics, and you have the Light's blessings and protection to follow your path. You will not be harmed, and you may do a great deal of good. Remember also to do healing for yourself; so many people (especially women) forget to do this.

Just for fun, try a midwives' pendulum technique for finding out the sex of an unborn child. With today's use of ultrasound, this information is given to the mother very early; we don't have to wait nine months anymore, but you might like to know before the medical system does. Do this test only after the seventh week of pregnancy, however, as before it, all your responses will be "female." In the embryo's seventh week, the hormone androgen activates if the baby is to be a boy. Unless and until this happens, the fetus registers female.

First, ask the mother-to-be if she wants to know, and only proceed with her permission. Using an absolutely energetically cleared pendulum, make contact with your Be-ing of the Highest Light and ask if she is willing to give you this information. If your pendulum says "yes," you may proceed. Your first request is to ask, "Is Karen pregnant?" "Yes." Next, for this request only, designate your "yes" response to mean "female" and your "no" response to be "male," and mentally tell your Be-ing of the Highest

Light that this is the code you wish to use. Hold the palm of your non-dominant hand a few inches in front of the mother's abdomen and ask, "What is the sex of the baby?" You will get your response and, sooner or later, be able to verify your accuracy. If your responses are both "yes" and "no," perhaps the children to come are twins, or you are not supposed to have the information yet.

You can do this with two questions instead of one, using your usual "yes" or "no" pendulum code. Ask, "Is the baby male?" "No." "Is the baby female?" "Yes." Next you might ask, "Is all well with the fetus?" The response will probably be "yes." If the response is "no," you can ask your Light Be-ing to help, and then ask if more is needed. Ask if the problem will right itself, as is usually the case. Ask if the midwife or doctor should be consulted. Do all this neutrally and calmly, and *don't scare the mother.* Ask your Be-ing of the Highest Light for help in assuring an easy pregnancy and the birth of a very healthy child. They will always help.

You can use your pendulum to discern the date the baby will be born. The mother will have been given a due date for delivery. With your pendulum ask, "Will the baby be born on the due date?" "No." They usually aren't, unless the birth is induced. Ask, "Will the baby be born before her due date?" "No." "Will she be born later than her due date?" "Yes." To find out how much later, ask, "One day?" "Two days?" and so on, until you find the birthday of the baby. Make a note of your information to verify later. The mother may want to know how many hours she will be in labor, or she may have other questions. Use your pendulum to find the answers.

There are a great many types of psychic and natural healing to choose from. I use Reiki and karmic release together, and usually suggest a gemstone or flower essence, a homeopathic remedy, an herb, or nutritional supplements—depending on what is needed by the person at the time. When a healing situation is presented to you, your first pendulum request might be to find out what healing modality would be best, or best to start with. Then, you can make a second request, asking for a "yes" for all of the other methods that it would be best to include. Name the types of healing work you are familiar with and get a "yes" or "no" for each. If there are going to be several methods, you might ask, "How many methods would be best to use for this person?" before listing them.

To find your answer to "how many," make your request and start counting. Say "one" and watch your pendulum's response—it will swing to "yes." "Two" is also a "yes." "Three," and it's still "yes." "Four," and the swing changes to "no." You will use three types of healing modalities; name the choices, one by one, asking for a "yes" or "no" with each. Three of the modalities will receive your pendulum's "yes" response. Sometimes the pendulum will register "no" until you say the correct number, switching then to "yes." You can also use a fan chart for this, writing the name of a healing method in each of its sections. (See diagram 6.) Hold your pendulum at the "hinge point," and first ask, "Which of these is the method to start with?" or, "Which is to be the primary healing method?" Then use your pendulum to determine the other modalities to add.

Once you decide upon a modality, there may be many choices within it. If you are looking for herbs for the flu or homeopathic remedies for a cold, for example, there are a number of these to choose from. Make a fan chart again, this time listing all of the possible herbs or all of the possible homeopathic remedies for the purpose. (See diagram 7.) This by no means takes the place of expertise or research into the modalities of herbalism or homeopathy, by the way. Sometimes, however, more than one remedy looks correct, and you want to know which is the most likely to help. With homeopathic remedies, there are often those that work best at each stage of a cold, and the one that works at first onset (usually Aconitum napellus, known as Aconite) will not work for the later, or end, stages of the dis-ease. You might use Kali bichromium (Kali bi) at the end, instead.

When designing your fan chart, be aware of this progression, and list your remedies accordingly. The first remedy at the bottom left might be Aconite for first onset; the remedies then follow in the order of the cold's progression, with Kali bi as the last item on the bottom right of the fan. If

DIAGRAM 6

HEALING METHODS FAN CHART

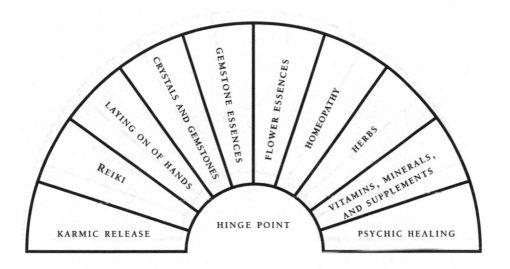

Use this fan chart to decide which healing modality (or modalities)
to use in a healing situation. Hold your pendulum at the hinge
point and ask, "Which of these is the method to start with?" Then
use your pendulum to determine other modalities to add.

DIAGRAM 7

HOMEOPATHY FOR COLDS FAN CHART[6]

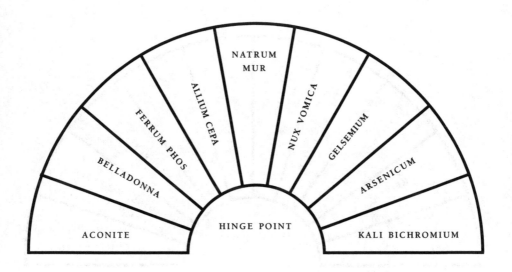

Use this fan chart to help you choose which homeopathic
remedy would help your cold. The question to ask is
"Which one?" The remedy that is optimal for you at early
onset may change as the cold progresses.

you are not proficient in the field, take the list of remedies from a good homeopathic guidebook. If you understand each remedy and how it works, you should be able to choose without a pendulum, as each has a different application for cold symptoms. I find, however, that pendulum use for choosing homeopathic remedies can be very helpful.

You can use lists to aid in your choice as well. Instead of making a fan chart, make a list of the possible healing methods, homeopathic remedies, and other remedies or herbs. Place your finger on the first item of the list asking, "Which do I need to help my cold?" Touch each item on the list with your finger, or a pointer held in your non-dominant hand, while using the cleared pendulum with your other (dominant) hand. Your pendulum will swing to "yes" at the item or items that are appropriate. Use a longer general herb list, containing herbs for a variety of uses, to determine which would be useful for your overall nutritional needs. Herbs are foods that heal dis-ease and support good health. Perhaps instead of, or along with, your herb for a cold, you could benefit from an immune building tea or extract. The longer general list has more choices, but you use it in the same way.

I use gemstones with almost every healing, suggesting a stone or quartz crystal as a beyond-physical vibrational aid to physical methods. I use my pendulum to determine what is needed. As with homeopathy, gemstones work on a nonphysical or beyond-physical level, but they have physical, emotional, mental, and spiritual effects. Use either a piece of the gemstone itself, placed in the aura by wearing it as jewelry or by carrying it in a pocket, or use a gemstone essence made with the energies of that stone. Essences are drops of water that are vibrationally charged with the gemstone and contain a small amount of brandy or vinegar as a preservative. They can also be made with the energies of flowers and these are wonderful healers too. Place a few drops of the essence on the tongue or in a glass of water to drink, and do this three or four times a day.

How to use gemstones and colors are basic healing skills. The colors of the gemstones match the chakra colors, and each chakra has a list of

DIAGRAM 8

GEMSTONES FOR THE CHAKRAS[7]

Root	Belly	Solar Plexus	Heart
Smoky Quartz	Carnelian	Topaz	Peridot
Black Tourmaline	Coral	Amber	Rose Quartz
Tourmaline	Red/Brown Agate	Citrine	Rhodochrosite
Quartz	Fire Agate	Tigereye	Pink Tourmaline
Obsidian	Orange Zircon	Golden Beryl	Green Tourmaline
Onyx	Orange Citrine	Malachite	Watermelon
Jet	Jacinth	Peridot	Tourmaline
Hematite	Brown Jasper	Yellow Jade	Emerald
Bloodstone	Phantom Calcite	Yellow Diamond	Green Jade
Garnet	Poppy Jasper	Chrysoberyl	Jadeite
Ruby	Wulfenite	Hawk's-eye	Nephrite
Red Jasper	Salmon Jade	Brazilianite	Green Aventurine
Rhodonite	Orange Sapphire	Apatite	Aquamarine
Magnetite	Orange Calcite	Sulphur	Turquoise
Lodestone	Orange Fluorite	Yellow Calcite	Chrysocolla
Red Zircon	Fire Opal	Green Tourmaline	Crysoprase
Black Star		Green Calcite	Green Quartz
Sapphire		Yellow Zircon	Kunzite
Red Fluorite		Green Zircon	Rhodonite
Red Jade		Yellow Tourmaline	Dolomite
		Yellow Sapphire	Pink Beryl
		Yellow Fluorite	Morganite
		Sphene	Pink Sapphire
		Yellow Barite	Green Sapphire
		Periclase	Rose Jade
		Malachite	Rose Coral
			Green Fluorite
			Pink Carnelian
			Rubelite

Throat	Brow	Crown/ Transpersonal Point
Aquamarine	Lapis Lazuli	Moonstone
Turquoise	Sodalite	Chalcedony
Chrysocolla	Blue Sapphire	Moss Agate
Amazonite	Blue Fluorite	Selenite
Blue Aventurine	Moonstone	Opal (Whitefire)
Blue Lace Agate	Chalcedony	Amethyst
Lapis Lazuli	Moss Agate	Clear Zircon
Sodalite	Azurite	Diamond
Blue Topaz	Star Sapphire	Rutile Quartz
Celestite	Dark Aquamarine	Clear Quartz
Blue Quartz	Blue Spinel	Alexandrite
Lazulite	Blue Zircon	Violet Garnet
Variscite	Zoisite	Iolite
Smithsonite	Lazulite	Violet Tourmaline
Gem Silica	Kyanite	Tanzanite
Eilat Stone	Aragonite	Ulexite
Malachite/Chrysocolla	Blue Tourmaline	Violet Fluorite
Malachite/Azurite	Malachite/Azurite	Pearl
Blue Zircon	Selenite	Sugilite
Blue Fluorite	Opal (White)	Violet Jade
Blue Chalcedony	Opal (Black)	Amethyst Quartz
	Fire Agate	Violet Zircon
	Desert Rose	Violet Sapphire

correspondences with organs, imbalances, and dis-eases. Gemstones operate by vibration, and if something is wrong in a chakra or an organ corresponding to it, the correct stone helps to right the imbalance by matching and harmonizing the vibration. If you are serious at learning healing, it is vital that you learn about the chakras and colors, what they mean, and how to use them. With that information, you will also have the uses of colored stones. Crystals can be programmed to carry any color or energy, and you can do color healing using light as well.

The list of gemstones for the chakras (see diagram 8) included here will help you know which gemstone or gemstone essence corresponds to each of the seven Kundalini chakras. Use this list with your pendulum to decide "which one?" as you have used lists before. If your pendulum and Light-being choose "carnelian," for example, you would either carry a piece of carnelian in your pocket, or ingest a few drops three times a day of carnelian gemstone essence. Use your pendulum to determine how long you need to use this energy. If you are using gemstones, they must be made and kept absolutely energetically cleared in the same way that your pendulums are. For more information on gemstone use and on using the chakras in healing, see my book *The Women's Book of Healing,* which is a complete course on the subject.

It is important that you know the location and colors of at least the seven primary Kundalini chakras, for they are vital information in psychic healing. (See diagram 9.) Most healers find this old information, like an infant's learning where her toes are. If you are new at healing, however, it's an important place to start.

Once you know the chakras, you can use the information your pendulum gains from assessing them for healing. The chakras are energy centers that reflect the health of all the bodies (physical, emotional, mental, and spiritual). We may be talking about physical healing here, but the chakras are energetic rather than physical, and they are used for the beyond-physical healing that may or may not affect the physical body.

DIAGRAM 9

THE KUNDALINI CHAKRAS[8]

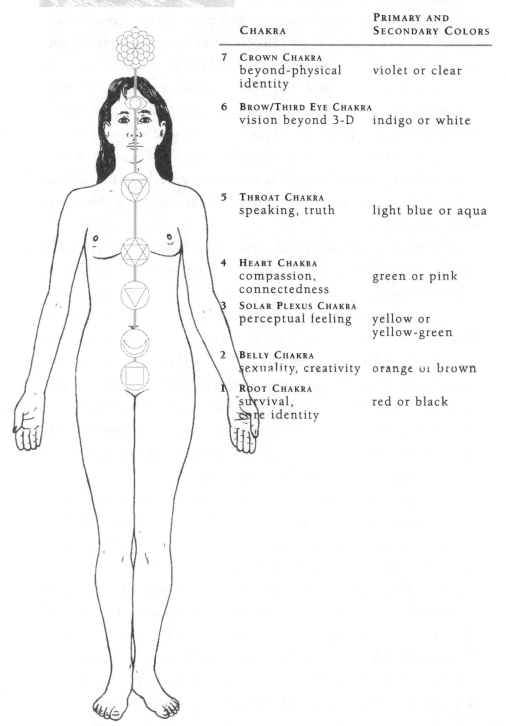

CHAKRA	PRIMARY AND SECONDARY COLORS
7 CROWN CHAKRA beyond-physical identity	violet or clear
6 BROW/THIRD EYE CHAKRA vision beyond 3-D	indigo or white
5 THROAT CHAKRA speaking, truth	light blue or aqua
4 HEART CHAKRA compassion, connectedness	green or pink
3 SOLAR PLEXUS CHAKRA perceptual feeling	yellow or yellow-green
2 BELLY CHAKRA sexuality, creativity	orange or brown
1 ROOT CHAKRA survival, core identity	red or black

The following information is how to use your pendulum to do a chakra assessment. You will assess another person in this example, as it is difficult to do it for yourself. Have the other person stand facing you without speaking. Both participants should be in an emotionally neutral state, with minds held quiet. Take your absolutely energetically cleared pendulum in your dominant hand, asking for the help of your Light-being. With your other hand, hold your palm a few inches away from the other person's body, over her Crown chakra at the top of her head. Notice your pendulum's swing. You have not made a request, but the pendulum will be swinging in a circle—notice whether it is a clockwise or counter-clockwise circle.

Move to the next chakra, placing your palm a few inches away from the person's Third Eye or Brow chakra (center forehead). Watch the pendulum's swing—it will reverse. Go to the next chakra, at the Throat. The pendulum reverses again. Do this moving down the chakras, over the Heart, Solar Plexus, Belly, and Root. The pendulum reverses each time. If something is imbalanced, constricted, or blocked in a chakra, however, the pendulum does not reverse, and it may go into a "no" response. In this case, asking your Be-ing of the Highest Light for help, hold your open palm steady over the chakra for two or three minutes. You will find that the chakra rights itself, and your pendulum's swing changes from "no" to "yes," moving into the proper directional swing.

Now try an aura assessment. The aura surrounds the energy bodies and physical body like multiple envelopes or layers of Light. If there are tears, holes, weak spots, imbalances, or other damage in these energetic envelopes, you are more prone to dis-ease, discomfort, the entrance of negative energies, or psychic attacks. Using your pendulum and open palm in the way you did before, first run your palm down the front, and then down the back and sides of the person's body. Hold your hand a few inches away without touching the person; it is the aura you are assessing, not the body itself. Move from head to feet. Do this very slowly, sensing the energy changes in your open hand and watching your pendulum's reactions. Your eyes and focus can move back and forth between the pendulum and your palm.

You will find that the aura feels springy and alive. At some spots over the body, however, the sensations change. Your hand may sense a cold or hot spot, a rough or wavy-feeling spot. The energy may seem to vibrate, or you may perceive what feels like a hole. With each of these sensations, ask your partner if there is or was any discomfort in the area. You may find that the hot spot you feel over her Third Eye is a headache, or the springy spot over her Belly chakra area is menstruation. You may find these sensations over a scar or where a bone was broken in the past, injuries long ago healed. What does your pendulum register over each of these spots?

Wherever you feel these areas of different energy, once you have asked the person if she knows what is there, try balancing the aura. Wait until you complete your assessment of the whole body, then put your pendulum down for a moment, asking that your Be-ing of the Highest Light stay with you and help you. Using both open palms this time, stroke the person's aura from head to feet and repeat for at least ten strokes. You can also "comb" the aura with curled fingers. Do the front, back, and sides this way. Now take your pendulum and go back to the spots that felt different before. You will find that they have "smoothed out" and match the rest of the aura. What does your pendulum register over each spot? Is it different from before the stroking and combing? Ask the person how she feels; she will like the sensations and feel better than she did, even if nothing serious had been wrong.

Also use the energy of the aura to help you find what vitamin, mineral, gemstone, or other remedy may be good for the person you are healing. You can do this for yourself too. You may have begun this with a list or fan chart, and the following is fine-tuning. To begin, take an example of the remedy in question—one capsule, the package or bottle, or the gemstone piece, and have the person hold it in her dominant hand. Take your pendulum in your dominant hand, and rest your other hand on the person's wrist, above where she is holding the remedy. Ask the pendulum and your

Light-being, "Will this remedy heal her headache?" The answer is "yes." (If it is "no," try a different remedy.) Your next question might be, "Is this the best possible remedy to heal her headache?" If the answer is "no," try other remedies until you find the right one.

Once you have the most optimal remedy, place it in the woman's hand again, asking, for example, "How many drops of this herb tincture does she need per dose?" Count until you get a "yes" for the correct number; start with ten drops, as she is likely to need from ten to thirty drops if the remedy is a liquid herb. Ask, "How many times will she need to take this remedy?" Your answer might be three or four times. Then ask how often to take it: "Does she need to take it once an hour?" "Does she need to take it every two hours?" "Every three hours?" Your pendulum tells you that she needs twenty drops of the remedy (always take herb tinctures in water, herbal tea, or juice), every three hours until she has taken four doses. At that point, if she still needs a remedy at all, do the process again.

If you are doing this work for yourself, hold the pendulum in your dominant hand and the item in your opposite hand. You can use this method in the health food store to choose vitamins, minerals, and supplements to take long-term, as well as for remedies you would take only while you have a specific discomfort or dis-ease. You can use it to choose which brand of a particular vitamin or remedy is the best for you. If you are doing this for yourself, hold the remedy package—or even touch it on the shelf—and ask about it with your pendulum. About every four months, I retest my daily vitamins, asking to see if I still need each of them or if there are dosage changes. In doing this, you may find that there are things you no longer need or that there are things to add.

You can use these methods in a gemstone or New Age store to choose crystals and stones that will help to balance your energy. Ask, "What stone do I need in my aura now?" Choose among several pieces of the same type, asking, "Which of these is best?" You may have to clear them, as you did when pendulum shopping, before you can get a valid answer. When my pendulum tells me "no" to a crystal or stone I want, I tell Brede, "It'll be cleared and dedicated as soon as we get home; with that in mind, would this be a good stone to buy?" Very often, the "no" changes to "yes." The stone or crystal was not recommended only because it needed cleansing. With that factor eliminated by your promise to purify and dedicate it, your answer may change. If it doesn't, obey your Light-being; she knows what you need and what is best for you.

I sometimes do a laying-on-of-stones healing, including it in a Reiki session, and as with most healing work, I use my pendulum. I ask the pendulum about each gemstone as I place it, to see if the stone should be included in the healing and where. Different stones match the vibrations and needs of different people and situations; everyone needs their own selection and placement. After choosing each gemstone and crystal, I ask, while holding it above the person's body where I think it should go, "Is this the best position for this stone?" In laying on of stones, crystals and gemstones are placed on top of each chakra, on the front of the physical body of a person who is lying on her back. This process is less easy to do for yourself if you are working alone, but it is possible. Match the colors of the stones with the colors of the chakras, and put the stones on the body where the chakras are located. You will need at least one gemstone or clear crystal for each chakra, and it's best to have more.

If you have several gemstones for each chakra color, you may find that some are to be used and some are not; use your pendulum to sort them. Your pendulum and Light-being may also place stones that are not specific for that chakra on it—a Third Eye stone on the Belly, for example. If you are using both colored gemstones and crystals, you will usually place the clear crystals between the chakras on the body. The person receiving the healing can hold them in her hand, and they may be placed on the floor above her head or below (or between) her feet. Let your pendulum guide you as to where each stone belongs in every healing.

You can also use your pendulum to tell you when the healing is complete and the stones are ready to be removed. This usually happens automatically, however, as they will just roll off the body when the healing is done. Wait for a while after this starts to happen, and ask if it's time to remove them all. Both participants will be laughing by that time. Before you begin the healing, be very certain that any stones used for healing have been absolutely energetically cleared (test with your pendulum for this). After ending the healing, the stones are to be cleansed again—every time without exception.

As you can see, there are a great many healing uses for pendulums. You will find them your most useful healing tool—after the help of your Light-being. You may find, when doing healing, that your Be-ing of the Highest Light will intervene, telling you to do some things and not do others, as she adds her own energy to the work. Ask for her help, as this is where the greatest of healing comes from. This is where the "miracle" healings begin to happen, though any healer will tell you that miracles happen in healing every day. Every healer has her stories, and an experienced healer has many of them.

When you add these techniques to working with the Lords of Karma for the karmic release of the sources of dis-ease and discomfort, you will see miracles indeed.

PENDULUMS AND KARMIC RELEASE

Karma is the essence of the concept that says, "What you do comes back to you." In this case, however, the "coming back" is over lifetimes. Souls are eternal and death is not the end of a human's or an animal's existence; it is only the end of one of numerous lives. We have experienced thousands of lifetimes, or incarnations, and not only on Earth. People did not originate on Earth, and we have had many of our incarnations on other planets. Karma also carries over from the between-life state, and from states of existence in which we are not in bodies. Our actions and the actions of others with regard to us survive the lifetime or lifetimes (or other states of existence) in which they originally occurred.

We can incarnate interchangeably as either male or female, but if you are human now, your incarnations have almost always been human. Dogs, cats, and horses can incarnate interchangeably; they may have had lifetimes as other kinds of animals too, and occasionally even as people. People and animals have karma, and so do Light-beings (who are also human, but who are on a higher evolutionary level than we are). In our many incarnations, we are expected to experience every facet and circumstance of living. That is the purpose of reincarnation: it would be impossible to experience everything in one lifetime, so we must have many lifetimes. Being in body, coming into incarnation, is the soul's evolutionary school. Our job in each incarnation is to be the best that we can be within the circumstances and experiences of each lifetime. Learning to love unconditionally is a major part of our evolutionary growth.

Many people believe that karma means "an eye for an eye," that what you do to someone else will return to you in precisely the same way—for example, that if you have been raped in this lifetime, you probably were a rapist in some past existence, and conversely, that the man who raped you was the person *you* raped in the past. While this can happen, it would be a rare occurrence. What is more likely is that if you have been raped in this lifetime, you have also been raped in past lifetimes, probably several of them, and it was probably the same rapist in different roles and relationships every time.

In another example, if you are an artist in this lifetime, you probably have been an artist in many other lifetimes, though maybe not the same kind of artist. You may be a painter now, but you could have been a pianist, architect, or singer in other incarnations. You have explored your life purpose, being an artist, in a variety of different ways. Each Be-ing has a life purpose that carries over from one incarnation to the next, and you will be drawn to that life purpose and helped to achieve it, again and again. You will be given opportunities to explore being an artist in every possible way and to serve humanity, the Earth, or the Light in doing so. This is another working out of karma, though this situation is usually called a "karmic gift" or "karmic reward," rather than karma itself. When we work at karmic release, these are things to have gratitude for, rather than to change.

In my understanding, the purpose of karma is to ensure the completion of both learning and healing. Karma is not punishment but is instead a lesson repeated until we "get it right." In the case of the woman who had been repeatedly raped, her lesson may be to finally and forever reject or refuse the rapist and reclaim her own power. In the case of the rapist, his karma may be to be stopped from being a predator, to be punished on Earth (or wherever else he did his crimes), or to lose forever his ability to hurt the woman he has raped or any other woman. One lesson for the rapist is that "crime doesn't pay," and to learn this, he may have to experience what he has wrought. In the bigger lesson, he may have to experience rape, or being preyed upon in other ways, before he understands through suffering what his actions did to others. Once he understands the lesson and changes himself so that he will never rape again, the karma is cleared.

For both the rapist and his victim, however, the damage to their spirits remains. Once the karma is fulfilled, the damage still has to be healed. If it is not, the woman's personality will express traits that lead to her being victimized again; the man may express personality traits that lead to his punishment continuing—he may become a prisoner who is raped by other men, for example. The learning of the lesson is not enough, because the damage leaves a pattern that returns again and again, repeating from lifetime to lifetime. This is the source of a karmic pattern, even if the karma itself has been fulfilled.

For the pattern to be released, ended so that there are no more perpetrators or victims, the damage has to be healed in each participant separately (though they are no longer karmically connected). This healing removes the source of the damage and allows the cycle to be completed. It's like a splinter being removed, so the festered and infected thumb can heal. Once this "splinter" is removed, the personality traits that cause the karma to continue are removed. The rapist will never rape again, and the woman who was raped will never be raped again. Both have hopefully learned enough about suffering so that they will never commit or suffer from rape again in any incarnation. And perhaps they will go on to help others to learn the same lessons.

Remember that we are all a part of the Collective Consciousness. When enough women refuse to be victimized, no one will be victimized again; when enough men learn respect for women and understand that rape is unthinkable, all rape will end. This change in the Collective Consciousness requires the critical mass that I have spoken of before. The goal of karma is that, both individually and collectively, humanity (and animals are not exempt) will evolve so that the horrors we commit against each other will end forever. I have used rape as an example, but it's so much more. The purpose is to end forever all the suffering that plagues all of life, or at least end as much of it as we can by amending our actions.

What about suffering? Not all suffering is caused by people intentionally hurting other people (or animals). Some seems quite random, like car accidents and dis-eases that kill and maim. No one caused this suffering or, at least, not by evil intent. There is no one to blame for a disease or a birth deformity, no one to blame for a fall or for being in the wrong place at the wrong time. Yet these things are karma as well. Evil and suffering are two different things, though evil causes some of our suffering. The difference between them is that evil causes suffering on purpose, but most suffering is not evil or done by evil intent. Nor is suffering as random as it sometimes seems. The purpose of suffering is to teach us compassion; we must experience every kind and way of life, including living in pain or being disabled or dying young from a virus. And we must learn to love even though we suffer. Evil must be overcome, and this can only be done through love—not by loving evil, but by loving ourselves and other people unconditionally and compassionately.

Until now, karma has been a process of long working out, over dozens of lifetimes and dozens of repetitions, until we release and heal each instance of it. The system seems to work, but the problem is that it's taking too long. The Collective Consciousness of the Earth isn't changing fast enough, and if our evolution as a whole doesn't accelerate, the Earth may not survive. We are in that dire a state. There had to be a solution, a way to rapidly clear karma for those incarnating on Earth and for the Earth itself. In 1995, I was given a very simple method for the clearing, healing, and release of karma; the idea was seeded on the planet, to see what we of Earth would do with such a gift.

I have been working with this process for eight years at the time of this writing, and teaching it to as many other people as are willing to learn and use it. It is the subject of four of my books so far (*We Are the Angels,*

Essential Energy Balancing, Reliance on the Light, and *Essential Energy Balancing II),* with at least one more *(Essential Energy Balancing III)* to come. If more of my work after that continues with karmic release work, I will not be surprised. It is that important a topic, with information vital to everyone. Along with Reiki, which I feel is its foundation discipline, karmic release is the most profound means of healing I have ever experienced or been privileged to teach.

The method is easy. Using a very simple formula, you make a request to the Lords of Karma for the release and healing of something that has meant suffering in your life. If you do the work as it is meant to be done, you will repeat the formula again and again, until *every* aspect and piece of karma and suffering in your life has been released and healed. The catch here is that you must make yourself aware of what's wrong in your life and be willing to change it, and you must do the work of making the requests. If you go all the way with this, you will achieve what New Age practitioners call Ascension and what in India is called Enlightenment. It is primarily a self-healing process.

There are levels of karma, as there are levels of other structures of our lives. Once you complete the release of all your Earth karma and the karma for our Solar System, you can work to release your karma at the levels of the Galaxy, Universe, Cosmos, and beyond, in turn. For your work of releasing the karma from all your lifetimes on Earth and everywhere else in this Solar System, including for the present lifetime, you will make your requests to the Lords of Karma. From the Galactic through the Cosmic levels, you will make your requests to Divine Director—the title of the Light-being in charge. But let's take it one step at a time.

The Lords of Karma are the keepers of karma for our Earth through Solar System levels. They are Light-beings who have been in body and have had many incarnations on Earth. They know Earth and how things work here thoroughly. They are also Ascended Masters, who have released all of their karma through the level of the Cosmos and beyond. They work for and under the direction of Nada, who is our Multi-Cosmic

Great Mother, and also sometimes under the direction of our First Mother, Eve, who is a First Source of the Light. Both of these Goddesses are our Creators.

The Lords of Karma act as advocates for those people who ask for karmic release. They are like the defense attorneys at a trial, with Nada as the Judge. Divine Director, who is a Presence of the Light on Nada's level, acts in the role of advocate before the Supreme Court. Both have authority to grant most of the karmic releases we ask for on their levels, but in some cases, where there is a question, Nada is the final Judge. These are Be-ings of the Highest Light to be approached and treated with deference and the greatest respect at all times. First Mother comes in where mercy and dispensation are called for, and at Her discretion. She may grant karmic releases for us.

The Lords of Karma come to us as a group (usually with a spokesperson), and Divine Director appears alone. There are eleven members in a Lords of Karma group, and they are assigned to one soul group. The Be-ings that come to you when you ask "to speak with the Lords of Karma" will probably be different from those who appear for your sister or your best friend who makes the same request. El Morya (who is Nada's Twin Flame) seems to have taken over the job of Divine Director now, since His predecessor has been recently reassigned. Any member of the Presences of the Light can grant Galactic-through-Cosmic karmic release requests, and if you ask "to speak with the Lords of Karma and Divine Director," a variety of individual Be-ings may appear in the Divine Director role. The job may be held for you by Kwan Yin, Jesus, Isis, Brede, or any of a number of other highest level Light-beings.

I am going to teach you these processes in such a way that you will be clearing both Earth-through-Solar System and Galactic (and eventually beyond) karma at once. In your requests, you will work with the Lords of Karma and Divine Director together. After you have completed all of your Earth-through-Solar System karmic releases, the request "to speak with the Lords of Karma and Divine Director" will bring in Divine

Director only, and the Lords of Karma will not appear. If your request is Earth-through-Solar System only in its reach, only the Lords of Karma will come when you ask to heal your karma. If your request is beyond the Solar System, even if you have not completed releasing all of your lower level karma, only Divine Director will come.

In order to do this on multiple levels at once, you must make a beginning karmic request of both the Lords of Karma and Divine Director to reconnect your full DNA complement (we will do this in a moment, so don't go ahead until I lead you through the process). This is needed to give you contact with the higher levels of the Light and to make your evolution—which is genetically transmitted, as is karma—possible. First, you need to learn to get in contact with, and meet, both your Lords of Karma group and the Be-ing of the Highest Light who will do Divine Director's work with you. Next, I will teach you how to do the process of karmic release. If you work very hard at releasing your karma, Nada or First Mother might introduce Herself to you. First walk before you fly, however.

When I teach this work, I ask my students to try to make contact with the Lords of Karma and Divine Director psychically, in the meditative altered state. For those who can't do it this way, I hand them a pendulum and teach them quickly to use it. The pendulum always works. I would like you to do the same—try it without the pendulum, and if you can work without it, do so. Otherwise, you can do this work entirely by pendulum. If you prefer to use the pendulum after you have made the first contact psychically, you may do so. The Lords of Karma and Divine Director are willing to work with you in either manner. However, if you can do the work without the pendulum, you may receive other sensory impressions and information that the pendulum's "yes-no-maybe" code can't offer. Understand also that when you do karmic release work with your pendulum it will be run by a different Be-ing of the Highest Light than usual.

The first time, or first few times, that you do this work, it is best to use the closed door and complete quiet of your meditative state. Once you get used to this work, you probably won't need it; you'll be able to easily switch into the altered state. For now, however, close the door and get quiet inside and out, and do a few minutes of the meditation exercises discussed previously in this book. When you are ready, have an absolutely energetically cleared pendulum in front of you (in case you need it), and ask "to speak with the Lords of Karma and Divine Director." With an open, ready mind, wait a few moments for response. If you are using your pendulum, it will swing to "yes." If you are not using your pendulum, you may have sensory impressions of them being there. You may see them, hear them, feel them, see a color or a Light, experience an emotion or a body sensation, or sense a presence.

Thank them for coming, then ask, as you did at the beginning of your pendulum work, "Please show me what a 'yes' response will be in my work with you." Wait a few moments and notice what you are given. Again this may be something you see, feel, or hear; you may hear someone say "yes." You may also perceive a color, burst of Light, sound of bells, a feeling of warmth in your heart, or any other variety of quiet and subtle responses. Once you understand the "yes," thank them. Then ask, "Please show me what a 'no' response will be in my work with you." Wait again and observe the result, and thank them when you have it. Sometimes a "no" is simply nothing happening. There can be no "maybes" in this work, only "yes" or "no." If you are unable to discern "yes" and "no," tell the Lords of Karma, and ask for their help; then try the above again.

If you still are unable to discern your "yes" and "no" responses psychically, pick up your pendulum. Ask, "Would the Lords of Karma and Divine Director be willing to run my pendulum for karmic release work?" The answer will always be "yes." You already are proficient in "yes" and "no" with a pendulum. If you get the "maybe" response, it usually means that you need to rephrase your question or add something, or that they want more information on a topic. Pay attention to the words that come into your head, and work quietly and be focused enough so that you can perceive them.

Once you are confident that the Lords of Karma and Divine Director (they'll work together in this) are willing to run your pendulum, or that you have psychic contact with them and you understand your "yes" and "no," make the following request in the exact words as I've written them. "I ask the Lords of Karma and Divine Director to clear, heal, reconnect, and fully activate the full complement of my DNA." There will be a "yes" or "no" response. If it is "yes," no more is needed, and there is no further process with this request.

If the response is "no," you must ask, "What do I need to do to have this?" Here, the psychic contact—the words that come into your mind—is important. They will tell you what to do and you must follow their directions. If you don't know how to follow their instructions, tell them, "I'm willing, but I don't know how; will you help me?" They will always agree to help and sometimes will agree to do what is necessary for you. Then, make your request again for the full complement of your DNA, using the precise words above. You will almost always get a "yes" this time. Thank them. You are now on the Ascension Path, if you weren't before.

Now you are ready to learn the process for releasing and healing your karma. This process releases and heals you of everything that is wrong in your life and that causes you suffering or harm. There are four categories of karmic release requests, and every request will fall into one of these four categories. Don't focus on the categories, however, but look at where you need the help. If the things hurting you seem impossible to heal (the things no one can do anything about), they are just the things to bring to the Lords of Karma and Divine Director for healing. If you thought you saw miracles in your healing work before, wait until you see what's coming now!

The categories of karma to make requests about include 1) dis-eases and health conditions on all levels; 2) relationships of all kinds; 3) life situations (such as poverty); and 4) character traits or habits you'd like to stop. You don't need to try to fit your requests into these categories—

they will fit automatically—but the categories will give you ideas of where to begin.

Dis-eases are always the first things that come to mind in karmic release work. It is best, however, to do some of the other requests first. Ask for healing for everything else that is immediately wrong in your life, since all of these things contribute to the dis-ease, whether you are aware of it or not. (In a moment, I will discuss what to do if you are refused a request.)

Relationships are most people's biggest karmic release category. Everyone in your life who has been difficult is included, from the boss who picks on you today to the babysitter who frightened you as a toddler. In the case of a negative relationship that has ended or that you wish to be ended, the request is to ask the Lords of Karma and Divine Director for "karmic release and healing from your relationship with [name]." If you wish to heal the relationship rather than end it, the request is for "karmic healing of the relationship with [name]." Make the requests about one person at a time. Requests to the Lords of Karma and Divine Director are phrased exactly like pendulum requests, and for the same reason—the limited possible response code (primarily "yes" or "no").

If the person you are asking for release from is someone in your life whom you want to never see again—your incest perpetrator, the punk who mugged you, your rapist—first make the request above and get the "yes." Then ask, "Is it for my best good to have karmic severance from this person?" If it's a "no," stop there. Only if the answer is "yes" may you make the next request, "I ask for karmic severance from this person." (These "yes" responses have a process that follows them; see below.)

For people in your life whom you love and with whom you want to have as optimal a relationship as possible, there is a different kind of relationship karmic work. Here the request would be to ask "for karmic healing and release from all that is negative in the relationship with [name]." This will heal a lot of karmic damage from the past, known and unknown, and prevent more. It will enhance the quality of the relationship and make it better.

As an example of karmic situations in your life that need healing, the classic one is poverty. You may ask "for karmic release from my poverty and all its sources and causes." Include "sources and causes" in every situational request, every request regarding a dis-ease, and every request regarding character traits. If poverty is an issue for you, consider asking for "the release of all outdated vows and oaths that are keeping me poor." At some time or another, we have all made vows of poverty that are still in effect until they are released, though they are no longer appropriate. There may be other kinds of outdated vows or oaths as well. You have no way of knowing what oaths you made in past lives, and it is best to clear those that no longer serve your best interest.

In the case of character traits, the request might be something like, "I ask for karmic release from saying 'well' at the beginning of all my sentences." This category includes any habits you wish to change. Ask the Lords of Karma and Divine Director "to grant me karmic release from my smoking addiction." (You will also have to do the work of quitting and sticking to quitting, of course.) Remember with every request to say "please" and "thank you" and to be grateful for what you are being given. Every one of these requests will change and heal your life in more ways than you now know.

Once you have made a request and it has been granted with your "yes" response, psychically or with the pendulum, use the process that follows. There are two parts. In the first section, you will need a "yes" for each phrase. The responses come quickly, and if you don't hear anything, it's probably been granted. If you receive a "no" to any part, ask if the item is needed, and if it's not, skip it and go to the next. If your psychic responses are unclear, check them on your pendulum, or do this process all by pendulum, making sure that the Lords or Karma and Divine Director are running the pendulum for you.

Part I reads

I ask for these healings through the Mind Grid Level,
      the DNA Level, the Karmic Contract Level, the Core
      Soul Level and Beyond, and through the Ascension Level;
From above and beyond my Moment of Self,
      to below and beyond the Core of the Earth,
      and everyone and everything in between;
And I ask to seal the cleared, healed energy
Unto the Light and Unto Protection forever.

If you receive a "no" for any of the above, ask if the relevant sections are needed, and if not, skip them and proceed. If you receive a "no" for any other reason than that it's not needed, you must release it as with other "no" responses. (How to do this is discussed below.)

Once you have a "yes" to all of the first part above, finish with the following, to which you also need a "yes." You can take this passage as all one request, and if you get a "yes" at the end, it's done. If you get a "no," however, you need to find which phrase is being refused. Part II is

I ask for these healings through all the levels and all the bodies,
All the lifetimes on Earth, and all other planets, including the present
      lifetime.
I ask to heal all the damage,
And bring the healing into the present,
NOW.

If you receive a "yes" for all of the above, the entire process is complete and karmic release has been granted. You will find your life changing profoundly, and every added karmic release will heal it further. Because the karma is not only released but also erased, you may find that by the time you finish both parts of the process, you don't remember what you are asking for. That's fine; it just works that way. You may also find that what you have asked to heal disappears, and you may not even remember that it was there before. You can do every step of this with your pendulum, and you can also use the pendulum to ask the Lords of Karma and Divine Director other questions about healing your karma. As long as you treat them with respect, you will be answered and helped in every way.

Some requests will be refused; your answer when you ask is "no." This is far from hopeless, as most "no" responses can be reversed or released. Never argue with the Lords of Karma or Divine Director. If you receive a "no" response, first ask whether the request is needed. Sometimes it's not. (I have students who think that they are terrible people, and when they ask to change, they are refused because they are not terrible at all!) If the request is needed and the answer is still a "no," your next request is, "What do I need to know or do to change this to a 'yes'?" You will hear, or know by it coming into your mind, what to do.

Sometimes you need to release another situation or past life, usually the lifetime where the karmic pattern originated—the first time it happened, or the first incident with the person. Whether you understand what you are being shown or not, do both parts of the process asking to release it. Once that's done, go back to your original question and ask it again. This time you will probably get a "yes." Do both parts of the process, and if it's "yes" all the way, you are finished and your request is granted.

Sometimes if you receive a "no," it's because there is other work that you need to do first. You might ask what that work is. If you don't know, make requests for what you *think* it is or what it might be. If that doesn't work, try rephrasing your question. There may be something that the Lords of Karma or Divine Director tell you to do. The one that comes up often is their instruction to "learn to love yourself." (Even if you don't know how to do this, agree to it and ask them for help.) If nothing else works, put the request aside and come back to it at another time, after you have done more work. Eventually, you will release the crucial piece of the puzzle, and your request will be granted. This often happens when asking to heal a dis-ease.

If you have not connected the full complement of your DNA (discussed earlier in this chapter), you will not be permitted to do the first part of the process. You will only be allowed do part II. This is because part I is Galactic and in the realm of Divine Director, and you cannot work with him without the DNA reconnection. According to science, on Earth we have two strands of DNA, but our full complement can be up to 181 strands (which science doesn't know about). These strands of DNA are other-dimensional and nonphysical; they will not appear in an electron microscope. The number of strands that will be connected for you depends upon how much karma you are willing to release. If you do the work, you can go all the way, and as you reach each new level, you will be guided in how to go further.

It requires the reconnection of twelve strands of DNA to complete your Ascension at the Earth-only level. It requires twenty-one strands for Solar System Ascension, thirty-eight to complete the Galaxy, fifty-five for Universal Ascension, and seventy-two strands of DNA for Ascension on the Cosmic Level. If, along with your karmic release work, you go through Essential Energy Balancing and reconnect thirty-eight or more DNA strands, you will bring in a Goddess or a God to join with you fully, as Brede has done with me. Ascension means that you are no longer required to reincarnate on the levels that you have completed; all your karma for those levels is released. None of this happens overnight, as each level requires a great many karmic release requests to complete it. There is no limit to your evolution, however, other than your willingness to work and to serve the Light.

If you wish to do your karmic release work using a pendulum, you may do so, though the psychic connection is optimal. Before you begin each and every session, make sure that the Lords of Karma and Divine Director are running your pendulum. Phrase your requests in the way that you have learned to phrase all of your pendulum requests, so that they can be answered fully by a "yes" or "no" response. (This is for all requests, whether you use the pendulum or not.) If you have done all the work of this book, you will find working with the Lords of Karma and Divine Director very easy to do. You will have learned how to run your pendulum optimally for the purpose. This purpose alone is the primary reason for this book, though all the other work is valid and will be useful to you in countless ways.

Karmic release will change your life. I can't begin to explain to you what a gift this work is; you will have to discover it for yourself by doing it. Use your pendulum to help you with karmic release and everyday uses, and you will have learned skills to keep for a lifetime. This book starts you in the right direction. Your own experience and practice with the information will make you proficient. If you choose to serve the Light in your life and work, you will be given every means of doing so, and every blessing will result

> Beltane Night
> May 1, 2003
> New Moon in Taurus

Notes

1. Greg Nielsen and Joseph Polansky, *Pendulum Power: A Mystery You Can See, a Power You Can Feel* (Rochester, VT: Destiny Books, 1987), 16. This is an excellent source for pendulum and dowsing history.

2. Richard Webster, *Dowsing for Beginners: The Art of Discovering: Water, Treasure, Gold, Oil, Artifacts* (St. Paul, MN: Llewellyn Publications, 1996), vi–xix.

3. Webster, *Dowsing for Beginners*, xxvii.

4. Nielsen and Polansky, *Pendulum Power*, 26.

5. Earlyne C. Chaney and Robert R. Chaney, *Astara's Book of Life: The Holy Breath in Man*, second degree, lesson four (Upland, CA: Astara, 1966), 23–24.

6. Remedies are derived from Stephen Cummings, F.N.P., and Dana Ullman, M.P.H., *Everybody's Guide to Homeopathic Medicines* (Los Angeles: Jeremy F. Tarcher, Inc., 1984), 71–75.

7. Diane Stein, *The Women's Book of Healing*, rev. ed. (Berkeley, CA: The Crossing Press, 2004), 271.

8. Diane Stein, *We Are the Angels: Healing Our Past, Present, and Future with the Lords of Karma* (Berkeley, CA: The Crossing Press, 1997), 29.

Suggested Reading

Askew, Stella. *How to Use a Pendulum.* Long Creek, SC: Tri-State Press, undated.

Chaney, Earlyne C., and Robert R. Chaney. *Astara's Book of Life: The Holy Breath in Man.* Upland, CA: Astara, 1966.

Cummings, Stephen, and Dana Ullman. *Everybody's Guide to Homeopathic Medicines.* Los Angeles: Jeremy F. Tarcher, Inc., 1984.

Fields, Anya. *Dowsing Dykes: How to Use a Pendulum as a Psychic and Healing Tool.* Milwaukee, WI: Crystal Revelations, 1982.

Fire Mountain Gems and Beads Jewelry Maker's Catalog. Fire Mountain Gems, One Fire Mountain Way, Grants Pass, OR 97526-2373. (800) 423-2319. Published yearly.

Longren, Sig. *The Pendulum Kit.* New York: Fireside Books, 1990.

Nielsen, Greg, and Joseph Polansky. *Pendulum Power: A Mystery You Can See, a Power You Can Feel.* Rochester, VT: Destiny Books, 1987.

Olson, Dale W. *Knowing Your Intuitive Mind: Advanced Pendulum Instruction and Applications.* Volume I. Eugene, OR: Crystalline Publications, 1991.

Ozaniec, Naomi. *Dowsing for Beginners.* London: Headway Books, Hodder & Stoughton, 1994.

Powell, Tag, and Judith Powell. *Taming the Wild Pendulum.* Pinellas Park, FL: Top of the Mountain Publishing, 1995.

Stein, Diane. *All Women Are Healers: A Comprehensive Guide to Natural Healing.* Berkeley, CA: The Crossing Press, 1990.

——. *Essential Reiki: A Complete Guide to the Ancient Healing Art.* Berkeley, CA: The Crossing Press, 1995.

——. *Psychic Healing with Spirit Guides and Angels.* Berkeley, CA: The Crossing Press, 1996.

——. *We Are the Angels: Healing Our Past, Present, and Future with the Lords of Karma.* Berkeley, CA: The Crossing Press, 1997.

——. *Essential Energy Balancing: An Ascension Process.* Berkeley, CA: The Crossing Press, 2000.

——. *Reliance on the Light: Psychic Protection with the Lords of Karma and the Goddess.* Berkeley, CA: The Crossing Press, 2001.

——. *Essential Energy Balancing II: Healing the Goddess.* Berkeley, CA: The Crossing Press, 2003.

——. *The Women's Book of Healing,* rev. ed. Berkeley, CA: The Crossing Press, 2004.

Thurnell-Read, Jane. *Geopathic Stress: How Earth Energies Affect Our Lives.* Shaftesbury, Dorset, UK: Element Books, 1995.

Webster, Richard. *Dowsing for Beginners: The Art of Discovering Water, Treasure, Gold, Oil, Artifacts.* St. Paul, MN: Llewellyn Publications, 1996.

Index